Covid-19

Editors

TIMOTHY D. HENRY
SANTIAGO GARCIA

HEART FAILURE CLINICS

www.heartfailure.theclinics.com

Consulting Editor
EDUARDO BOSSONE

Founding Editor
JAGAT NARULA

April 2023 • Volume 19 • Number 2

ELSEVIER

1600 John F. Kennedy Boulevard • Suite 1800 • Philadelphia, Pennsylvania, 19103-2899

http://www.theclinics.com

HEART FAILURE CLINICS Volume 19, Number 2
April 2023 ISSN 1551-7136, ISBN-13: 978-0-443-18358-4

Editor: Joanna Gascoine
Developmental Editor: Jessica Cañaberal

Heart Failure Clinics (ISSN 1551-7136) is published quarterly by Elsevier Inc., 360 Park Avenue South, New York, NY 10010-1710. Months of publication are January, April, July, and October. Business and editorial offices: 1600 John F. Kennedy Boulevard, Suite 1800, Philadelphia, PA 19103-2899. Periodicals postage paid at New York, NY, and additional mailing offices. Subscription prices are USD 291.00 per year for US individuals, USD 629.00 per year for US institutions, USD 100.00 per year for US students and residents, USD 315.00 per year for Canadian individuals, USD 729.00 per year for Canadian institutions, USD 331.00 per year for international individuals, USD 729.00 per year for international institutions, and USD 100.00 per year for Canadian and foreign students/residents. To receive student and resident rate, orders must be accompanied by name of affiliated institution, date of term, and the *signature* of program/residency coordinator on institution letterhead. Orders will be billed at individual rate until proof of status is received. Foreign air speed delivery is included in all *Clinics* subscription prices. All prices are subject to change without notice. **POSTMASTER:** Send address changes to *Heart Failure Clinics*, Elsevier Health Sciences Division, Subscription Customer Service, 3251 Riverport Lane, Maryland Heights, MO 63043. **Customer Service: 1-800-654-2452 (US and Canada). From outside of the US and Canada, call 314-447-8871. Fax: 314-447-8029. For print support, E-mail: JournalsCustomerService-usa@elsevier.com. For online support, E-mail: JournalsOnlineSupport-usa@elsevier.com.**

Reprints. For copies of 100 or more of articles in this publication, please contact the Commercial Reprints Department, Elsevier Inc., 360 Park Avenue South, New York, NY 10010-1710. Tel.: 212-633-3874; Fax: 212-633-3820; E-mail: reprints@elsevier.com.

Heart Failure Clinics is covered in *MEDLINE/PubMed (Index Medicus)*.

Contributors

CONSULTING EDITOR

EDUARDO BOSSONE, MD, PhD, FCCP, FESC, FACC
Department of Public Health, "Federico II"
University of Naples, Naples, Italy

EDITORS

TIMOTHY D. HENRY, MD
The Christ Hospital Heart and Vascular
Institute, The Carl and Edyth Lindner Center for
Research and Education, The Christ Hospital,
Cincinnati, Ohio, USA

SANTIAGO GARCIA, MD
Minneapolis Heart Institute, Minneapolis,
Minnesota, USA; The Christ Hospital,
Cincinnati, Ohio, USA

AUTHORS

M. CHADI ALRAIES, MD
DMC Harper University Hospital, Detroit,
Michigan, USA

SHY AMLANI, MD
William Osler Health System, Brampton,
Ontario, Canada

HERBERT D. ARONOW, MD, MPH
Lifespan Cardiovascular Institute, Department
of Medicine, Division of Cardiology, The
Warren Alpert Medical School of Brown
University, Providence, Rhode Island, USA

AKSHAY BAGAI, MD, MHS
Terrence Donnelly Heart Centre, St. Michael's
Hospital, University of Toronto, Toronto,
Ontario, Canada

ALIREZA BAGHERLI, MD
Windsor Regional Hospital, Windsor, Ontario,
Canada

MURTAZA BHARMAL, MD
Department of Cardiology, University of
California Irvine Medical Center, Irvine,
California, USA

ANNA E. BORTNICK, MD, PhD, MSc
Albert Einstein College of Medicine,
Department of Medicine, Division of
Cardiology, Division of Geriatrics, Montefiore
Medical Center, Bronx, New York,
USA

NICHOLE BOSSON, MD, MPH, NRP, FAEMS
Assistant Medical Director, Los Angeles
County Emergency Medical Services Agency,
Sante Fe Spring, California, USA; EMS
Fellowship Director and Faculty, Department of
Emergency Medicine, Harbor-UCLA Medical
Center, Torrance, California, USA; Clinical
Associate Professor of Emergency Medicine,
David Geffen School of Medicine at UCLA, Los
Angeles, California, USA

SUSAN CHENG, MD, MPH, MMSc
Department of Cardiology, Smidt Heart
Institute, Cedars-Sinai Medical Center, Los
Angeles, California, USA

AUN-YEONG CHONG, MD
University of Ottawa Heart Institute, Ottawa,
Ontario, Canada

NICK CURZEN, BM (Hons), PhD, FRCP
Faculty of Medicine, University of
Southampton and University Hospital
Southampton NHS Foundation Trust,
Southampton, United Kingdom

ABDULLA A. DAMLUJI, MD, PhD, MPH
Associate Professor of Medicine (Cardiology),
Johns Hopkins School of Medicine, Inova
Center of Outcomes Research, Falls Church,
Virginia, USA

LAURA DAVIDSON, MD
Northwestern University Feinberg School of
Medicine, Chicago, Illinois, USA

LAURA DE MICHIELI, MD
Department of Cardiovascular Diseases, Mayo
Clinic, Rochester, Minnesota, USA;
Department of Cardiac, Thoracic, Vascular
Sciences and Public Health, University of
Padova, Padova, Italy

PAYAM DEHGHANI, MD
Prairie Vascular Research Inc, Regina,
Saskatchewan, Canada

KYLE DIGRANDE, MD
Department of Cardiology, University of
California Irvine Medical Center, Irvine,
California, USA

JOSEPH E. EBINGER, MD, MS
Department of Cardiology, Smidt Heart
Institute, Cedars-Sinai Medical Center, Los
Angeles, California, USA

MATTEO FRONZA, MD
Department of Medical Imaging, Toronto
General Hospital, Peter Munk Cardiac Center,
University Health Network (UHN), University of
Toronto, Toronto, Ontario, Canada

MOHAMED GABR, MD
Albert Einstein College of Medicine,
Department of Medicine, Division of
Cardiology, Montefiore Medical Center, Bronx,
New York, USA

**CHRIS P. GALE, MB BS, BSc (Hons), PhD,
FRCP**
Leeds Institute of Cardiovascular and
Metabolic Medicine, Leeds Institute for Data
Analytics, University of Leeds, Department of
Cardiology, Leeds Teaching Hospitals NHS
Trust, Leeds, United Kingdom

NIKHIL R. GANGASANI, MPH
Inova Center of Outcomes Research, Inova
Heart and Vascular Institute, Falls Church,
Virginia, USA; Johns Hopkins School of
Medicine, Baltimore, Maryland, USA; Medical
College of Georgia, Augusta, Georgia, USA;
Northside Hospital Cardiovascular Institute,
Atlanta, Georgia, USA

SANTIAGO GARCIA, MD
Minneapolis Heart Institute, Minneapolis,
Minnesota, USA; The Christ Hospital,
Cincinnati, Ohio, USA

NIMA GHASEMZADEH, MD
Georgia Heart Institute, Gainesville, Georgia,
USA

KARI GORDER, MD
The Christ Hospital Heart and Vascular
Institute, Cincinnati, Ohio, USA

CINDY L. GRINES, MD
Inova Center of Outcomes Research, Inova
Heart and Vascular Institute, Falls Church,
Virginia, USA; Johns Hopkins School of
Medicine, Baltimore, Maryland, USA; Medical
College of Georgia, Augusta, Georgia, USA;
Northside Hospital Cardiovascular Institute,
Atlanta, Georgia, USA

RAVITEJA R. GUDDETI, MD
Minneapolis Heart Institute Foundation,
Minneapolis, Minnesota, USA

KATE HANNEMAN, MD, MPH
Department of Medical Imaging, Toronto
General Hospital, Peter Munk Cardiac Center,
University Health Network (UHN), University of
Toronto, Toronto, Ontario, Canada

TIMOTHY D. HENRY, MD
The Christ Hospital Heart and Vascular
Institute, The Carl and Edyth Lindner Center for
Research and Education, The Christ Hospital,
Cincinnati, Ohio, USA

SULEMAN ILYAS, MD
Division of Cardiology, The Warren Alpert
Medical School of Brown University,
Providence, Rhode Island, USA

ALLAN S. JAFFE, MD
tDepartment of Cardiovascular Diseases,
Department of Laboratory Medicine and
Pathology, Mayo Clinic, Rochester, Minnesota,
USA

ROHAN KANKARIA, BS
Albert Einstein College of Medicine, Montefiore
Medical Center, Bronx, New York, USA

NAVIN K. KAPUR, MD
Tufts Medical Center, Boston, Massachusetts,
USA

SHARMILA KHULLAR, MD
Department of Laboratory Medicine and
Pathobiology, University of Toronto,
Laboratory Medicine Program, University
Health Network, Toronto, Ontario, Canada

NATHAN KIM, MD
Department of Internal Medicine, Northeast
Georgia Health System, Gainesville, Georgia,
USA

**THOMAS A. KITE, BMEDSCI (HONS), BM,
BS, MRCP**
Department of Cardiovascular Sciences and
the NIHR Leicester Biomedical Research
Centre, Glenfield Hospital, University of
Leicester and University Hospitals of Leicester
NHS Trust, Leicester, United Kingdom

ARAVIND KOKKIRALA, MD
United States Department of Veterans Affairs
Providence VA Medical Center, Providence,
Rhode Island, USA

ANDREW LADWINIEC, MA, MD, FRCP
Department of Cardiovascular Sciences and
the NIHR Leicester Biomedical Research
Centre, Glenfield Hospital, University of
Leicester and University Hospitals of Leicester
NHS Trust, Leicester, United Kingdom

DAVID W. LOUIS, MD
Lifespan Cardiovascular Institute, Department
of Medicine, Division of Cardiology, The
Warren Alpert Medical School of Brown
University, Providence, Rhode Island, USA

MINA MADAN, MD, MHS
Schulich Heart Centre, Sunnybrook Health
Sciences Centre, Toronto, Ontario, Canada

MAMAS A. MAMAS, MD, DPhil
Professor of Cardiovascular Medicine, Keele
Cardiovascular Research Group, Keele
University, Keele, United Kingdom;
Department of Cardiology Thomas Jefferson
University, Philadelphia, Pennsylvania, USA;

Institute of Population Health, University of
Manchester, Manchester, United Kingdom

CONSTANTIN A. MARSCHNER, MD
Department of Medical Imaging, Toronto
General Hospital, Peter Munk Cardiac Center,
University Health Network (UHN), University of
Toronto, Toronto, Ontario, Canada;
Department of Radiology, University Hospital,
LMU Munich, Munich, Germany

KESHAV R. NAYAK, MD
Scripps Mercy Hospital, San Diego, California,
USA

**SUSIL PALLIKADAVATH, MBChB (Hons),
BSc (Hons)**
Department of Cardiovascular Sciences and
the NIHR Leicester Biomedical Research
Centre, Glenfield Hospital, University of
Leicester and University Hospitals of Leicester
NHS Trust, Leicester, United Kingdom

AKASH PATEL, MD
Department of Cardiology, University of
California Irvine Medical Center, Irvine,
California, USA

VALERIYA POZDNYAKOVA, BS
F. Widjaja Foundation Inflammatory Bowel and
Immunobiology Research Institute, Cedars-
Sinai Medical Center, Los Angeles, California,
USA

ZAHRA RAISI-ESTABRAGH, MD, PhD, NIHR
Clinical Lecturer, William Harvey Research
Institute, NIHR Barts Biomedical Research
Centre, Queen Mary University, Barts Heart
Centre, St Bartholomew's Hospital, Barts
Health NHS Trust, London, United Kingdom

MARWAN SAAD, MD, PhD
Lifespan Cardiovascular Institute, Department
of Medicine, Division of Cardiology, The
Warren Alpert Medical School of Brown
University, Providence, Rhode Island, USA

YADER SANDOVAL, MD
Department of Cardiovascular Diseases, Mayo
Clinic, Rochester, Minnesota, USA

CRISTINA SANINA, MD
Albert Einstein College of Medicine,
Department of Medicine, Division of
Cardiology, Montefiore Medical Center, Bronx,
New York, USA

JACQUELINE SAW, MD
Vancouver General Hospital, Vancouver,
British Columbia, Canada

MICHAEL A. SEIDMAN, MD, PhD
Department of Laboratory Medicine and
Pathobiology, University of Toronto,
Laboratory Medicine Program, University
Health Network, Toronto, Ontario, Canada

JAY S. SHAVADIA, MD
Royal University Hospital, Saskatchewan
Health, University of Saskatchewan,
Saskatoon, Saskatchewan, Canada

DAVID M. SHAVELLE, MD
MemorialCare Heart and Vascular Institute,
Long Beach Medical Center, Long Beach,
California, USA

KIRSTEN E. SHAW, MD
Department of Graduate Medical Education,
Abbott Northwestern Hospital, Minneapolis,
Minnesota, USA

JYOTPAL SINGH, MSc
Prairie Vascular Research Inc, Regina,
Saskatchewan, Canada

TIMOTHY D. SMITH, MD
The Christ Hospital Heart and Vascular
Institute, Cincinnati, Ohio, USA

**PAALADINESH THAVENDIRANATHAN, MD,
SM**
Department of Medical Imaging, Division of
Cardiology, Peter Munk Cardiac Centre,
Toronto General Hospital, University Health
Network (UHN), University of Toronto, Toronto,
Ontario, Canada

FELIPE SANCHEZ TIJMES, MD
Department of Medical Imaging, Toronto
General Hospital, Peter Munk Cardiac Center,

University Health Network (UHN), University of
Toronto, Toronto, Ontario, Canada;
Department of Medical Imaging, Clinica Santa
Maria, Universidad de los Andes, Santiago,
Chile

JACOB A. UDELL, MD, MPH
Division of Cardiology, Peter Munk Cardiac
Centre, Toronto General Hospital, University
Health Network (UHN), Cardiovascular
Division, Women's College Hospital, University
of Toronto, Toronto, Ontario, Canada

SHILPA VIJAYAKUMAR, MD
Lifespan Cardiovascular Institute, Department
of Medicine, Division of Cardiology, The
Warren Alpert Medical School of Brown
University, Providence, Rhode Island, USA

RACHEL M. WALD, MD
Department of Medical Imaging, Division of
Cardiology, Peter Munk Cardiac Centre,
Toronto General Hospital, University Health
Network (UHN), University of Toronto, Toronto,
Ontario, Canada

BRITTANY WEBER, MD, PhD
Carl J. and Ruth Shapiro Cardiovascular
Center, Brigham and Women's Hospital,
Boston, Massachusetts, USA

JOSE WILEY, MD, MPH
Albert Einstein College of Medicine,
Department of Medicine, Division of
Cardiology, Montefiore Medical Center, Bronx,
New York, USA

MEHMET YILDIZ, MD
The Christ Hospital, Cincinnati, Ohio, USA

WESLEY YOUNG, BS
The Christ Hospital Heart and Vascular
Institute, Cincinnati, Ohio, USA

Contents

The Coronavirus 2019 (COVID-19) pandemic, caused by the Severe Acute Respiratory Syndrome Coronavirus-2 (SARS-CoV-2) virus, has resulted in unprecedented morbidity and mortality worldwide. While COVID-19 typically presents as viral pneumonia, cardiovascular manifestations such as acute coronary syndromes, arterial and venous thrombosis, acutely decompensated heart failure (HF), and arrhythmia are frequently observed. Many of these complications are associated with poorer outcomes, including death. Herein we review the relationship between cardiovascular risk factors and outcomes among patients with COVID-19, cardiovascular manifestations of COVID-19, and cardiovascular complications associated with COVID-19 vaccination.

Myocardial injury is common in patients with COVID-19 and is associated with an adverse prognosis. Cardiac troponin (cTn) is used to detect myocardial injury and assist with risk stratification in this population. SARS-CoV-2 infection can play a role in the pathogenesis of acute myocardial injury due to both direct and indirect damage to the cardiovascular system. Despite the initial concerns about an increased incidence of acute myocardial infarction (MI), most cTn increases are related to chronic myocardial injury due to comorbidities and/or acute nonischemic myocardial injury. This review will discuss the latest findings on this topic.

We herein summarize currently available and clinically relevant information regarding the human immune responses to SARS-CoV-2 infection and vaccination, in relation to COVID-19 outcomes with a focus on acute respiratory distress syndrome (ARDS) and myocarditis.

The novel SARS-CoV-2 has directly and indirectly impacted patients with acute coronary syndrome (ACS). The onset of the COVID-19 pandemic correlated with an abrupt decline in hospitalizations with ACS and increased out-of-hospital deaths. Worse outcomes in ACS patients with concomitant COVID-19 have been reported, and acute myocardial injury secondary to SARS-CoV-2 infection is recognized. A rapid adaptation of existing ACS pathways has been required such that overburdened health care systems may manage both a novel contagion and existing illness. As SARS-CoV-2 is now endemic, future research is required to better define the complex interplay of COVID-19 infection and cardiovascular disease.

outcome after both out-of-hospital and in-hospital cardiac arrest were reduced. Direct effects of the COVID-19 illness combined with indirect effects of the pandemic on patient's behavior and health care systems contributed to these changes. Understanding the potential factors offers the opportunity to improve future response and save lives.

Mechanical Complication of Acute Myocardial Infarction Secondary to COVID-19 Disease   241

Abdulla A. Damluji, Nikhil R. Gangasani, and Cindy L. Grines

The aggressive inflammatory response to COVID-19 can result in airway damage, respiratory failure, cardiac injury, and multiorgan failure, which lead to death in susceptible patients. Cardiac injury and acute myocardial infarction (AMI) secondary to COVID-19 disease can lead to hospitalization, heart failure, and sudden cardiac death. When serious collateral damage from tissue necrosis or bleeding occurs, mechanical complications of myocardial infarction and cardiogenic shock can ensue. While prompt reperfusion therapies have decreased the incidence of these serious complications, patients who present late following the initial infarct are at increased for mechanical complications, cardiogenic shock, and death. The health outcomes for patients with mechanical complications are dismal if not recognized and treated promptly. Even if they survive serious pump failure, their CICU stay is often prolonged, and their index hospitalization and follow-up visits may consume significant resources and impact the health care system.

Myocarditis Following COVID-19 Vaccination   251

Constantin A. Marschner, Kirsten E. Shaw, Felipe Sanchez Tijmes, Matteo Fronza, Sharmila Khullar, Michael A. Seidman, Paaladinesh Thavendiranathan, Jacob A. Udell, Rachel M. Wald, and Kate Hanneman

Myocarditis is an established but rare adverse event following administration of messenger RNA–based coronavirus disease 2019 (COVID-19) vaccines and is most common in male adolescents and young adults. Symptoms typically develop within a few days of vaccine administration. Most patients have mild abnormalities on cardiac imaging with rapid clinical improvement with standard treatment. However, longer term follow-up is needed to determine whether imaging abnormalities persist, to evaluate for adverse outcomes, and to understand the risk associated with subsequent vaccination. The purpose of the review is to evaluate the current literature related to myocarditis following COVID-19 vaccination, including the incidence, risk factors, clinical course, imaging findings, and proposed pathophysiologic mechanisms.

Cardiovascular Health Care Implications of the COVID-19 pandemic   265

Zahra Raisi-Estabragh and Mamas A. Mamas

The coronavirus disease 2019 (COVID-19) pandemic has challenged the capacity of health care systems around the world, including substantial disruptions to cardiovascular care across key areas of health care delivery. In this narrative review, we examine the implications of the COVID-19 pandemic for cardiovascular health care, including excess cardiovascular mortality, acute and elective cardiovascular care, and disease prevention. Additionally, we consider the long-term public health consequences of disruptions to cardiovascular care across both primary and secondary care settings. Finally, we review health care inequalities and their driving factors, as highlighted by the pandemic, and consider their importance in the context of cardiovascular health care.

HEART FAILURE CLINICS

SERIES OF RELATED INTEREST

Cardiology Clinics
http://www.cardiology.theclinics.com/
Cardiac Electrophysiology Clinics
https://www.cardiacep.theclinics.com/
Interventional Cardiology Clinics
https://www.interventional.theclinics.com/

THE CLINICS ARE AVAILABLE ONLINE!
Access your subscription at:
www.theclinics.com

Preface
Cardiovascular Effects of COVID-19

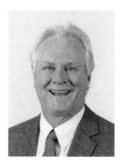

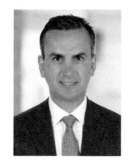

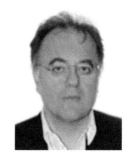

Timothy D. Henry, MD, FACC, MSCAI

Santiago Garcia, MD, FACC, FSCAI

Eduardo Bossone, MD, PhD, FCCP, FESC, FACC

Editors

The COVID-19 pandemic has had a dramatic impact on the care of patients with cardiovascular disease throughout the world. COVID-19 has a myriad of direct effects on the myocardium, vasculature, and coagulation cascade, related to the proinflammatory and prothrombotic effects of the virus, leading to an increased risk of myocardial infarction, stroke, deep venous thrombosis, and pulmonary emboli within the first 2 to 4 weeks of contracting the disease (**Fig. 1**).[1–4]

Patients with heart failure constitute a subgroup of patients at high risk of complications from COVID-19.[5,6] Preexisting heart failure is associated with increased mortality in patients hospitalized with COVID-19. Worsening functional heart failure class has been associated with increased duration of hospitalization and escalation of therapies leading to increased mortality.[5,6] Similarly, 3% to 25% of patients developed left-ventricular dysfunction after admission from COVID-19. The overall mortality for hospitalized heart failure patients with COVID-19 was between 4% and 40%. Possible mechanisms of COVID-19 and heart failure include effects of proinflammatory cytokine storm in patients with COVID-19 affecting the myocardium, direct myocardial injury, such as myocarditis, coronary thrombosis, late presentations of acute myocardial infarction, and acute respiratory failure leading to myocardial supply, demand mismatch leading to oxidative stress and damage to the cardiomyocytes. The role of mRNA vaccines, as potential triggers of myocarditis, is also an important consideration, particularly in young men.

The indirect effects of the pandemic in terms of disruption of health care processes and pathways of care have been as dramatic.[2,7–9] Public health measures designed to mitigate the spread of the virus, such as lockdowns, cancellation or deferral of elective procedures, in person appointments, and restrictive visitation policies, resulted in patients' reluctance to obtain both elective and emergent medical care. This resulted in a reduction in the number of patients with ST-segment elevation myocardial infarction (STEMI) presenting to hospitals throughout the world and significant delays in those who did arrive.[9] This led to a dramatic increase in mortality for patients with non-STEMI and STEMI with a higher rate of out-of-hospital cardiac arrest, cardiogenic shock, and late complications of acute myocardial infarction, including heart failure.[8] These deleterious effects on cardiovascular outcomes have been documented in patients with and without COVID. In

Heart Failure Clin 19 (2023) xi–xiii
https://doi.org/10.1016/j.hfc.2023.02.001
1551-7136/23/© 2023 Published by Elsevier Inc.

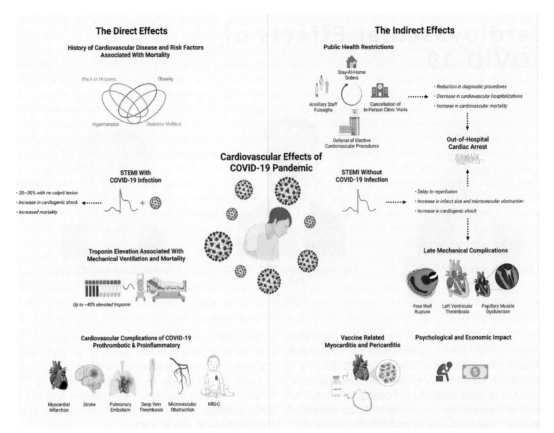

Fig. 1. The direct and indirect effects of COVID-19 on cardiovascular disease. (*From* Henry TD, Kereiakes DJ. The direct and indirect effects of the COVID-19 pandemic on cardiovascular disease throughout the world. Eur Heart J. 2022 Mar 14;43(11):1154-1156. https://doi.org/10.1093/eurheartj/ehab782. PMID: 34791131; PMCID: PMC8690059.)

addition, there have been significant economic and psychologic impacts on patients throughout the world.

We believe this outstanding collection of articles regarding both the direct and the indirect effects of the COVID-19 pandemic will help us to improve the care of cardiovascular patients.

Timothy D. Henry, MD, FACC, MSCAI
The Carl and Edyth Lindner Center
for Research and Education
2139 Auburn Avenue
Cincinnati, OH 45219, USA

Santiago Garcia, MD, FACC, FSCAI
Structural Heart Program
The Carl and Edyth Lindner Center for
Research and Education at The Christ Hospital
2139 Auburn Avenue
Cincinnati, OH 45219, USA

Eduardo Bossone, MD, PhD, FCCP, FESC, FACC
Department of Public Health
"Federico II" University of Naples
Via Pansini, 5
80131 Naples, Italy

E-mail addresses:
Tim.Henry@thechristhospital.com (T.D. Henry)
santiagogarcia@me.com (S. Garcia)
eduardo.bossone@unina.it (E. Bossone)

REFERENCES

1. Madjid M, Safavi-Naeini P, Solomon SD, et al. Potential effects of coronaviruses on the cardiovascular system: a review. JAMA Cardiol 2020;5:831–40.
2. Gupta A, Madhavan MV, Sehgal K, et al. Extrapulmonary manifestations of COVID-19. Nat Med 2020;26: 1017–32.

3. Henry TD, Kereiakes DJ. The direct and indirect effects of the COVID-19 pandemic on cardiovascular disease throughout the world. Eur Heart J 2022;43:1154–6.

4. Garcia S, Dehghani P, Grines C, et al. Initial findings from the North American COVID-19 Myocardial Infarction Registry. J Am Coll Cardiol 2021;77:1994–2003.

5. Bhatt AS, Jering KS, Vaduganathan M, et al. Clinical outcomes in patients with heart failure hospitalized with COVID-19. JACC Heart Fail 2021;9:65–73.

6. Alvarez-Garcia J, Lee S, Gupta A, et al. Prognostic impact of prior heart failure in patients hospitalized with COVID-19. J Am Coll Cardiol 2020;76:2334–48.

7. Gluckman TJ, Bhave NM, et al. 2022 ACC expert consensus decision pathway on cardiovascular sequelae of COVID-19 in adults: myocarditis and other myocardial involvement, post-acute sequelae of SARS-CoV-2 infection, and return to play: a report of the American College of Cardiology Solution Set Oversight Committee. J Am Coll Cardiol 2022;79:1717–56.

8. Nadarajah R, Wu J, Hurdus B, et al. The collateral damage of COVID-19 to cardiovascular services: a meta-analysis. Eur Heart J 2022;43:3164–78.

9. Garcia S, Albaghdadi MS, Meraj WM, et al. Reduction in ST-segment elevation cardiac catheterization laboratory activations in the United States during COVID-19 pandemic. J Am Coll Cardiol 2020;75:2871–2.

The Cardiovascular Manifestations of COVID-19

David W. Louis, MD[a,b], Marwan Saad, MD, PhD[a,b],
Shilpa Vijayakumar, MD[a,b], Suleman Ilyas, MD[b], Aravind Kokkirala, MD[c],
Herbert D. Aronow, MD, MPH[a,b,*]

KEYWORDS

- COVID-19 • Acute coronary syndrome • Thrombosis • Heart failure

KEY POINTS

- Pre-existing cardiovascular comorbidities significantly increase the risk of hospitalization and death secondary to COVID-19 infection.
- Cardiovascular manifestations of COVID-19 include acute coronary syndromes, arterial and venous thrombosis, acutely decompensated heart failure (HF), myopericarditis, stress-induced cardiomyopathy, and arrhythmia.
- COVID-19 vaccination-related cardiac adverse events have been reported, but these occur far less frequently than cardiovascular and other complications related to SARS-CoV-2 infection.

INTRODUCTION

The Coronavirus 2019 (COVID-19) pandemic, caused by the Severe Acute Respiratory Syndrome Coronavirus-2 (SARS-CoV-2) virus, has resulted in unprecedented morbidity and mortality worldwide. Since March 2020, there have been more than 80 million cases, 4 million hospital admissions, and approximately 980,000 deaths in the US alone.[1] The US Food and Drug Administration's (FDA) emergency use authorization (EUA) of 3 COVID-19 vaccines (Pfizer BioNTech, Moderna, and Janssen/Johnson & Johnson) has led to more than 500 million vaccinations, with 83% of the US population partially and 71% fully vaccinated at the time of writing.[2] COVID-19 vaccines offer immense protection, both in reducing the contraction of disease and in reducing the risk of severe illness requiring hospitalization. The risks of testing positive and of dying from COVID-19 are 4 and 15 times higher in unvaccinated individuals than among those who are vaccinated, respectively.

While COVID-19 typically presents as viral pneumonia, cardiovascular manifestations including acute myocardial injury and acute coronary syndromes (ACS), venous and arterial thrombosis, cardiomyopathy, and arrhythmia have all been observed (**Fig. 1**). Herein we review the relationship between cardiovascular risk factors and COVID-19 outcome, and the cardiovascular manifestations of COVID-19.

ASSOCIATION BETWEEN CARDIOVASCULAR COMORBIDITIES AND COVID-19 OUTCOMES

Observational studies published early in the pandemic have suggested that underlying cardiovascular comorbidities and risk factors, including coronary artery disease (CAD), heart failure (HF), hypertension (HTN), and diabetes mellitus (DM),

This article originally appeared in Cardiology Clinics, Volume 40, Issue 3, August 2022.
[a] Lifespan Cardiovascular Institute, 593 Eddy Street, RIH APC 730, Providence, RI 02903, USA; [b] Department of Medicine, Division of Cardiology, Alpert Medical School of Brown University, 222 Richmond Street, Providence, RI 02903, USA; [c] United States Department of Veterans Affairs Providence VA Medical Center, 830 Chalkstone Avenue, Providence, RI 02908, USA
* Corresponding author. 593 Eddy Street, RIH APC 730, Providence, RI 02903.
E-mail address: Herbert.Aronow@Lifespan.org

Mechanisms of Injury and Cardiovascular Complications of COVID-19

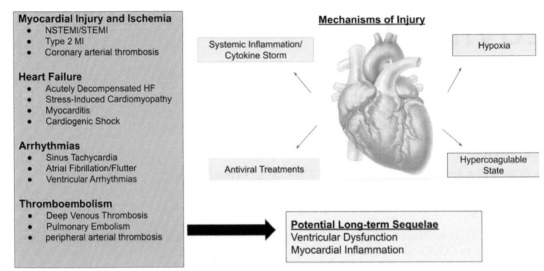

Fig. 1. Cardiovascular manifestations of COVID-19. Patients with COVID-19, particularly those with underlying co-morbidities, are at significant risk for both acute and postrecovery cardiovascular complications.

were associated with worse outcomes in patients diagnosed with COVID-19 infection.[3–6] In an observational study of 1590 patients admitted with COVID-19 in China, DM [hazard ratio (HR) 1.59 (95% confidence interval (CI):: 1.03–2.45), $P = .037$], HTN [HR 1.58 (95% CI: 1.07–2.32), $P = .022$], and the presence of 2 or more preadmission comorbidities [HR 2.59 (95% CI: 1.61–4.17), $P < .001$] significantly increased the risk of intensive care unit (ICU) admission, invasive ventilation, or death.[3] In an analogous observational study of 5700 patients hospitalized with COVID-19 in the New York City area, 56% had HTN, 42% were obese, 11% had CAD, and 7% had underlying HF.[6] In a large multicenter database analyzing 132,312 patients with a history of HF who were hospitalized from April 2020 to September 2020%, 6.4% were hospitalized with COVID-19 infection. Nearly 1 in 4 patients with HF hospitalized with COVID-19 died during hospitalization.[7] Other cohort studies have also correlated an increased likelihood of ICU level of care[4] and worse survival[5] among those with overt cardiovascular disease at baseline.

CARDIOVASCULAR MANIFESTATIONS OF COVID-19
Myocardial Injury

The Fourth Universal Definition of Myocardial Infarction defines acute myocardial injury as a rise and/or fall of cardiac troponin with at least one value > 99th percentile of the upper reference limit without otherwise meeting the criteria for an acute myocardial infarction (symptoms of myocardial ischemia, new ischemic ECG changes, development of pathologic Q waves, imaging evidence suggesting loss of viable myocardium, or the identification of coronary thrombus).[8] Given that myocardial injury can occur in the setting of acute stressors such as infection, hypoxemia, anemia, hypotension/shock, acute kidney injury, and congestive HF, it is unsurprising that patients admitted with COVID-19 are frequently found to have myocardial injury.[9–11] The prevalence of myocardial injury in patients hospitalized with COVID-19 ranges from 5% to 38%, with an overall crude prevalence of approximately 20%.[12]

Myocardial injury occurs with relatively higher frequency in patients with COVID-19 who have underlying cardiovascular disease. In a retrospective case series of 187 patients from Wuhan City, China hospitalized with COVID-19, patients with elevated Tn-T levels were more likely to have HTN, CAD, or cardiomyopathy at baseline, compared to those without elevated troponin.[9] Similarly, in a cohort of 416 patients admitted with COVID-19, cardiac injury was associated with chronic HTN, DM, CAD, and cerebrovascular disease. In both of the above reports, patients with myocardial injury were more likely to present with abnormal laboratory results including higher elevations in white blood cell counts, C-reactive protein, procalcitonin, N-terminal pro-B-type natriuretic peptide, and creatinine, and with lower levels of platelets and albumin, all of which suggests that those with myocardial injury are more critically ill.[9,10]

The presence of myocardial injury in those with COVID-19 has also been associated with a significant increase in mortality. Guo and colleagues[9] observed markedly higher in-hospital adverse events including death, acute respiratory distress syndrome (ARDS), malignant arrhythmias, acute coagulopathy, and acute kidney injury in patients with elevated Tn-T levels compared with patients with normal Tn-T. Shi and colleagues[10] similarly found that patients with myocardial injury experienced higher rates of mortality, both from time of symptom onset and from index admission date. Additionally, in a study of 179 patients with COVID-19 pneumonia, elevated troponin-I (Tn-I) was a predictor of mortality.[11] The presence of myocardial injury in patients hospitalized for COVID-19 suggests critical systemic illness, and these patients fare poorly even if the criteria for myocardial infarction are absent.

Acute Coronary Syndromes

Acute viral infections, such as SARS-CoV-2, are associated with the activation of inflammatory, prothrombotic, and procoagulant cascades,[13] which likely play an important role in the increased risk of ACS through coronary plaque instability and thrombosis.[13] At the onset of the pandemic, significant reductions in hospitalizations for chest pain and ACS[14,15] and an increased incidence of out-of-hospital cardiac arrest were noted.[16] Although uncertain, these observations were likely in part related to containment measures implemented to help mitigate the spread of COVID-19 and patient fears of nosocomial COVID-19 infection.

Among patients who did present to hospitals with ST-elevation myocardial infarction (STEMI) during this time, comorbid conditions, including dyslipidemia, DM, and tobacco use disorder, were more common, and patients were more likely to present with cardiogenic shock.[17] While primary PCI remained the gold standard for the treatment of ACS, strained hospital resources, perceived risk to catheterization laboratory personnel, and system delays negatively impacting door-to-balloon time prompted conversations about the use of fibrinolytics for patients presenting with STEMI.[18,19] In a large observational study evaluating in-hospital mortality in patients hospitalized with STEMI, fibrinolytics were used more frequently as reperfusion therapy in patients with COVID-19 than in patients without COVID-19 (0.2% vs 1.9%; $P < .001$), but their use was still much less common than that of primary percutaneous coronary intervention.[20]

Patients with STEMI and COVID-19 have increased in-hospital mortality. In a retrospective analysis of 28,189 patients with STEMI in China between December 27, 2019 – February 20, 2020, a higher likelihood of in-hospital mortality [odds ratio (OR): 1.21; (95% CI: 1.07–1.37); $P = .003$] was observed in those with versus without COVID-19.[21] Similarly, in a retrospective cohort study of 80,449 US patients from the Vizient Clinical Database admitted between January 1, 2019 and December 31, 2020, rates of in-hospital mortality among patients propensity matched on the likelihood of COVID-19 were higher in those who were COVID-19 positive than COVID-19 negative both for out-of-hospital (15.2% vs 11.2%, $P = .007$) and in-hospital STEMI (78.5% vs 46.1%; $P < .001$).[20] Additionally, the composite outcome of death, stroke, or MI and the composite outcome of death or stroke were both more frequently observed in the in- and out-of-hospital STEMI cohorts.[20] Reassuringly, the mortality rate among patients with STEMI without COVID-19 were similar during the pandemic when compared with 2019, suggesting that alterations in systems of care were not to blame for the increased mortality.[20]

Thrombotic Complications

Complex interactions between SARS-CoV-2 and platelets, viral-mediated microvascular trauma, proinflammatory cytokine release, and endothelial dysfunction results in micro- and macrovascular complications.[22–24] Markers of systemic inflammation and hypercoagulability are elevated in patients with severe COVID-19, particularly those requiring ICU level of care,[4,25] and an elevated D-dimer has been shown to independently predict the likelihood of developing an arterial thrombotic event.[26] Furthermore, baseline elevations and up-trending D-dimer levels throughout a patient's hospital course have been associated with increased mortality risk.[4,5,27]

Studies have noted a variable but elevated incidence of venous thromboembolism (VTE) among patients hospitalized with COVID-19.[27–31] The risk of VTE seems to be significantly higher in hospitalized than ambulatory patients with COVID-19.[29] In a meta-analysis of 48 studies with a total pooled sample of 18,093 patients, the overall pooled incidence of VTE, deep vein thrombosis (DVT) and pulmonary embolism (PE) was 17.0% (95% CI: 13.4–20.9), 12.1% (95% CI: 8.4–16.4%), and 7.1% (95% CI: 5.3–9.1%), respectively.[32] The incidence of VTE is significantly higher among patients cared for in the ICU compared with a medical ward (27.9% vs 7.1%).[32] Other venous thromboses have been reported, including catheter-associated thrombosis,[31] renal replacement therapy (RRT) filter thrombosis,[33] and portal and mesenteric vein thromboses.[34]

Arterial thromboembolism including acute ischemic stroke, ACS, acute limb ischemia (ALI), mesenteric, renal, and splenic infarcts have all been documented in patients with COVID-19.[26,27,33,35,36] In a study of patients with COVID-19 presenting with STEMI, those with COVID-19 were more likely to have multivessel coronary thrombosis, stent thrombosis and more likely to require adjunctive glycoprotein IIb/IIIa inhibitor agents, aspiration thrombectomy, and multivessel PCI compared with patients without COVID-19.[37] Furthermore, grade 2 to 3 myocardial blush suggesting improved myocardial perfusion was more common in patients without than with COVID-19.[37] An observational study from the Lombardi region of Italy noted a significant rise in cases of ALI during a 3-month period compared with the prior year (16.3% vs 1.8%, $P < .001$).[38] Notable predictors of ALI included greater than 50% lung involvement on CT scan, elevated D-dimer, and low fibrinogen.[26] Furthermore, in-hospital death was significantly higher in patients with COVID-19 and an acute thrombotic event than in those with COVID-19 but without a thrombotic event (40% vs 16.2%, $P = .002$); relatedly, those with both a thrombotic event and COVID-19 had a higher in-hospital mortality rate than those with a thrombotic event in the absence of concomitant COVID-19 infection (40% vs 3.1%, $P < .001$).[26]

Acute ischemic stroke secondary to large vessel occlusion has also been documented in patients hospitalized with COVID-19.[36] In a retrospective, self-controlled case series of 5119 patients with COVID-19 in a Danish hospital, the incidence of ischemic stroke was approximately 10 times higher (incidence ratio 12.9 [95% CI: 7.1–23.5; $P < .001$]) when compared with patients during a pre–COVID-19 control time interval.[36] A higher rate of stroke has been observed in hospitalized patients with COVID-19 than influenza.[39] Importantly, however, in a retrospective study of 8163 patients, only 1.3% with symptomatic COVID-19 and 1.0% of asymptomatic COVID-19 developed an acute ischemic stroke, suggesting that while the relative risk of stroke is significantly increased, the absolute risk remains low.[40] Nonetheless, in this cohort, in-hospital mortality was significantly higher following acute ischemic stroke in those with COVID-19 than without COVID-19 (19.4% vs 6.2%, $P < .0001$%).[40]

Heart Failure and Cardiogenic Shock

Patients with chronic HF are particularly vulnerable to SARS-CoV-2 infection. Early in the pandemic, reductions in ED visits and hospitalizations for acute decompensated HF were noted.[41,42] Despite these reductions, chronic HF remained

an important risk factor for admission in patients with COVID-19.[43]

In-hospital complications including death were more frequently observed in patients with underlying HF admitted for COVID-19.[44,45] In a study of 6439 patients admitted with COVID-19, the risk of ICU admission [adjusted OR: 1.71; (95% CI: 1.25–2.34); $P = .001$], intubation and mechanical ventilation [adjusted OR: 3.64; (95% CI: 2.56–5.16); $P < .001$, and in-hospital mortality [adjusted OR: 1.88; (95% CI: 1.27–2.78); $P = .002$] were significantly higher in patients with than without pre-existing HF.[44] Notably, risk was similar irrespective of whether patients had HF with reduced ejection fraction (HFrEF) or HF with preserved ejection fraction (HFpEF).[44] In a meta-analysis of 18 studies, mortality in patients with both COVID-19 and pre-existing HF was significantly higher than in patients with COVID-19 without pre-existing HF [OR: 3.46; (95% CI: 2.52–4.75); $P < .001$].[45]

Myocarditis with or without pericardial involvement (myopericarditis) is an uncommon but well-documented complication of viral infection and can result in hospitalization, HF, arrhythmia, and sudden death.[46] Myocarditis has been reported secondary to influenza[47] and Middle Eastern respiratory syndrome coronavirus (MERS-CoV)[48] in previously healthy patients. Pathologic mechanisms responsible for viral myocarditis are hypothesized to include a postviral autoimmune reaction, antigenic mimicry, and direct immune injury with cytokine storm.[49,50] Presenting signs and symptoms of acute myocarditis are nonspecific (dyspnea, chest pain, palpitations, peripheral edema, presyncope/syncope) and can delay diagnosis. In patients with suspected acute myocarditis, diagnostic strategies should include the assessment of cardiac biomarkers, inflammatory markers, and echocardiographic evaluation of ventricular function.

There have been many reports of COVID-19-associated myocarditis since the onset of the pandemic.[51] Using a large, US hospital-based administrative database from more than 900 hospitals, the Center for Disease Control (CDC) assessed the association between COVID-19 and myocarditis and observed that patients with COVID-19 were approximately 15 times more likely to be diagnosed with myocarditis than those without COVID-19.[52] COVID-19-related myocarditis seems to have a male predominance and can occur irrespective of comorbid conditions.[53] Furthermore, myocardial injury, reductions in left ventricular (LV) systolic function, pericardial effusions with or without tamponade physiology, and cardiogenic shock have all been documented.[53,54]

Stress-induced ("Takotsubo") cardiomyopathy with apical ballooning has also been documented in patients with COVID-19. Case reports have described this complication in both male and female patients with and without pre-existing comorbidities.[55] Proposed etiologic mechanisms are similar to those of acute myocarditis including an exaggerated immune response with cytokine storm, overstimulation of the sympathetic nervous system, and microvascular dysfunction.[55] Documented complications of stress-induced cardiomyopathy include LV dysfunction, cardiogenic shock, LV thrombus, dynamic LV outflow tract obstruction, QT prolongation, atrial and ventricular arrhythmias, pericardial effusions, and death.[56]

Cardiac Arrhythmias

Both atrial and ventricular arrhythmias are commonly observed in patients with COVID-19. Palpitations have been reported as the presenting symptom in 10% of patients,[57] and sinus tachycardia has been documented as the most common cardiac rhythm disturbance, likely as a physiologic compensation mechanism to acute illness.[58] An early report from China noted that 17% of their total cohort and 44% of patients requiring ICU level of care had documented arrhythmia[4]; however, in a larger cohort of 700 patients admitted to a Pennsylvania hospital with COVID-19, no cases of heart block, sustained ventricular tachycardia (VT), or ventricular fibrillation (VF) were noted, and only 9 episodes of clinically significant bradyarrhythmia resulting in hypotension, 25 incidents of atrial fibrillation requiring amiodarone and diltiazem, and 10 nonsustained VT episodes were observed.[59]

Atrial fibrillation and flutter (AF) are the most commonly encountered cardiac dysrhythmias in the United States[60] and are associated with an increased risk of stroke, transient ischemic attack (TIA), and other arterial emboli. Both the risk of mortality[61] and thromboembolic complications[62] are higher among patients with COVID-19 who also have preexisting AF. In a large systematic review and analysis of 19 studies totaling 21,653 patients hospitalized with COVID-19, the pooled prevalence of AF was 11%. In subgroup analysis, patients ≥ 60 years old exhibited a 2.5-fold higher prevalence, and patients with severe COVID-19 had a 6-fold higher prevalence of AF compared with younger and less critically ill patients, respectively.[63] The use of pre-admission oral anticoagulation (OAC) with either a direct oral anticoagulant (DOAC) or vitamin K antagonist (VKA) in patients with AF admitted with COVID-19 has been associated with lower composite rates of in-hospital death or thrombotic events, and less severe COVID-19. These observations,

while hypothesis generating, may suggest that subclinical and clinical thrombosis are prevented by the use of pre-admission OAC.[64]

The initial EUA of hydroxychloroquine for the treatment of COVID-19 sparked concern regarding the risk of QT prolongation and Torsade de Pointes. However, subsequent studies observed modest QT/QTc prolongation, with low rates of major ventricular arrhythmia rates and no-arrhythmia-related deaths. Furthermore, in retrospective studies[65] and prospective randomized controlled trials,[66] the use of hydroxychloroquine with or without azithromycin did not improve clinical status or mortality. As a result, hydroxychloroquine has fallen out of favor.

COVID-19 VACCINES

COVID-19 vaccine-induced complications have been described following the release of COVID-19 and adenoviral-vector vaccines. Cases of presumed vaccine-induced pericarditis and myocarditis confirmed by cardiac MRI have been observed in otherwise healthy adolescents and young adults within days of vaccination.[67,68] Large observational studies subsequently confirmed a very low incidence of vaccine-associated myocarditis, seen more commonly among White males.[69,70] Other cardiovascular complications after COVID-19 adenoviral vector vaccines (eg, AstraZeneca and Janssen/Johnson & Johnson) have been reported including immune thrombotic thrombocytopenia (TTS),[71] cerebral venous sinus thrombosis,[71] VTE, TIA and stroke, acute myocardial infarction, arrhythmia, and large-vessel vasculitis including Kawasaki disease.[72] Nonetheless, these complications are rare and occur much less commonly than following SARS-CoV-2 infection.[73]

LONG-TERM CONSEQUENCES OF COVID-19

The long-term cardiovascular effects of SARS-CoV-2 infection have not been fully established and remain a focus of ongoing studies. Using a national cohort of 153,760 patients from the US Department of Veterans Affairs, Xie and colleagues[74] observed that prior infection with COVID-19 was associated with an increased incidence of cerebrovascular disorders, dysrhythmias, pericarditis, myocarditis, ischemic heart disease, HF, and thromboembolic events 1 year after infection, when compared with both contemporary and historical control groups. Notably, the increase in cardiovascular complications was observed regardless of whether patients had a history of prior cardiovascular disease and regardless of whether they required hospitalization or ICU admission during active infection. Nevertheless, the severity of initial SARS-CoV-2 infection was associated with the likelihood of postinfection cardiovascular complications.[74]

Long-COVID, a term used to describe persistent symptoms after recovery from acute COVID-19 infection, is also being closely investigated. Symptoms including fatigue, sleep disturbances, nonspecific chest pain, dyspnea, and gastrointestinal upset have all been reported. Quantitative findings supportive of multi-organ involvement have been documented, including abnormalities in liver enzymes, acute kidney injury, reductions in circulating T and B lymphocytes, and elevated troponin.[75] Long-term follow-up of patients with long-COVID is needed to better understand the consequences of COVID-19 infection.

SUMMARY

The COVID-19 pandemic has resulted in significant morbidity and mortality worldwide. There has been increasing progress in understanding and defining cardiovascular manifestations of COVID-19 illness. Patients hospitalized with COVID-19, particularly those with underlying cardiovascular comorbidities, are at high risk for developing serious cardiovascular manifestations such as acute myocardial injury and ACS, HF and cardiogenic shock, systemic thromboembolism, and arrhythmia. A thorough understanding of these complications may better prepare clinicians and improve patient outcomes.

CLINICS CARE POINTS

- Patients with cardiovascular risk factors and overt cardiovascular disease are more likely to be hospitalized, have more severe disease, and experience poorer outcomes in the setting of COVID-19.
- COVID-19 vaccination is essential among patients with cardiovascular risk factors and overt disease to ameliorate these risks.[76]

DISCLOSURE

The authors have nothing to disclose.

REFERENCES

1. CDC - Cases, Deaths, & Testing. Available at: https://covid.cdc.gov/covid-data tracker/#cases_casesper100klast7days. Accessed February 25, 2022.
2. CDC – COVID Data Tracker. COVID-19 vaccinations in the United States. Available at: https://covid.cdc.gov/covid-data-tracker/#vaccinations_vacc-total-admin-rate-total. Acessed February 25, 2022.
3. Guan W jie, hua Liang W, Zhao Y, et al. Comorbidity and its impact on 1590 patients with COVID-19 in China: a nationwide analysis. Eur Respir J 2020; 55(5):2000547.
4. Wang D, Hu B, Hu C, et al. Clinical characteristics of 138 hospitalized patients with 2019 novel coronavirus–infected pneumonia in wuhan, China. JAMA 2020;323(11):1061–9.
5. Zhou F, Yu T, Du R, et al. Clinical course and risk factors for mortality of adult inpatients with COVID-19 in Wuhan, China: a retrospective cohort study. Lancet 2020;395(10229):1054–62.
6. Richardson S, Hirsch JS, Narasimhan M, et al. Presenting characteristics, comorbidities, and outcomes among 5700 patients hospitalized with COVID-19 in the New York City area. JAMA 2020; 323(20):2052–9.
7. Bhatt AS, Jering KS, Vaduganathan M, et al. Clinical outcomes in patients with heart failure hospitalized with COVID-19. JACC Heart Fail 2021;9(1):65–73.
8. Thygesen K, Alpert JS, Jaffe AS, et al. Fourth universal definition of myocardial infarction (2018). J Am Coll Cardiol 2018;72(18):2231–64.
9. Guo T, Fan Y, Chen M, et al. Cardiovascular Implications of fatal outcomes of patients with Coronavirus disease 2019 (COVID-19). JAMA Cardiol 2020;5(7):1–8.
10. Shi S, Qin M, Shen B, et al. Association of cardiac injury with mortality in hospitalized patients with COVID-19 in Wuhan, China. JAMA Cardiol 2020; 5(7):802–10.
11. Du RH, Liang LR, Yang CQ, et al. Predictors of mortality for patients with COVID-19 pneumonia caused by SARS-CoV-2: a prospective cohort study. Eur Respir J 2020;55(5):2000524.
12. Bavishi C, Bonow RO, Trivedi V, et al. Acute myocardial injury in patients hospitalized with COVID-19 infection: a review. Prog Cardiovasc Dis 2020; 63(5):682–9.
13. Sandoval Y, Januzzi JL, Jaffe AS. Cardiac troponin for the diagnosis and risk-stratification of myocardial injury in COVID-19: JACC review topic of the week. J Am Coll Cardiol 2020;76(10):1244–58.
14. Filippo OD, D'Ascenzo F, Angelini F, et al. Reduced rate of hospital admissions for ACS during Covid-19 outbreak in northern Italy. N Engl J Med 2020; 383(1).
15. Helal A, Shahin L, Abdelsalam M, et al. Global effect of COVID-19 pandemic on the rate of acute coronary syndrome admissions: a comprehensive review of published literature. Open Heart 2021;8(1): e001645.
16. Lai PH, Lancet EA, Weiden MD, et al. Characteristics associated with out-of-hospital cardiac arrests

and resuscitations during the novel Coronavirus disease 2019 pandemic in New York City. JAMA Cardiol 2020;5(10):1154–63.

17. Garcia S, Dehghani P, Grines C, et al. Initial findings from the North American COVID-19 myocardial infarction registry. J Am Coll Cardiol 2021;77(16):1994–2003.

18. Wang N, Zhang M, Su H, et al. Fibrinolysis is a reasonable alternative for STEMI care during the COVID-19 pandemic. J Int Med Res 2020;48(10). https://doi.org/10.1177/0300060520966151.

19. Daniels MJ, Cohen MG, Bavry AA, et al. Reperfusion of ST-segment–elevation myocardial infarction in the COVID-19 era. Circulation 2020;141(24):1948–50.

20. Saad M, Kennedy KF, Imran H, et al. Association between COVID-19 diagnosis and in-hospital mortality in patients hospitalized with ST-segment elevation myocardial infarction. JAMA 2021;326(19):1940–52.

21. Xiang D, Xiang X, Zhang W, et al. Management and outcomes of patients with STEMI during the COVID-19 pandemic in China. J Am Coll Cardiol 2020;76(11):1318–24.

22. Page EM, Ariëns RAS. Mechanisms of thrombosis and cardiovascular complications in COVID-19. Thromb Res 2021;200:1–8.

23. Miesbach W, Makris M. COVID-19: coagulopathy, risk of thrombosis, and the rationale for anticoagulation. Clin Appl Thromb Hemost 2020;26. https://doi.org/10.1177/1076029620938149.

24. Goshua G, Pine AB, Meizlish ML, et al. Endotheliopathy in COVID-19-associated coagulopathy: evidence from a single-centre, cross-sectional study. Lancet Haematol 2020;7(8):e575–82.

25. Guan WJ, Ni ZY, Hu Y, et al. Clinical characteristics of Coronavirus disease 2019 in China. N Engl J Med 2020;382(18).

26. Fournier M, Faille D, Dossier A, et al. Arterial thrombotic events in adult inpatients with COVID-19. Mayo Clin Proc 2021;96(2):295–303.

27. Bilaloglu S, Aphinyanaphongs Y, Jones S, et al. Thrombosis in hospitalized patients with COVID-19 in a New York City health system. JAMA 2020;324(8):799–801.

28. Middeldorp S, Coppens M, Haaps TF van, et al. Incidence of venous thromboembolism in hospitalized patients with COVID-19. J Thromb Haemost 2020;18(8):1995–2002.

29. Roubinian NH, Dusendang JR, Mark DG, et al. Incidence of 30-day venous thromboembolism in adults tested for SARS-CoV-2 infection in an integrated health care system in Northern California. JAMA Intern Med 2021;181(7):997–1000.

30. Lodigiani C, Iapichino G, Carenzo L, et al. Venous and arterial thromboembolic complications in COVID-19 patients admitted to an academic hospital in Milan, Italy. Thromb Res 2020;191:9–14.

31. Klok FA, Kruip MJHA, van der Meer NJM, et al. Incidence of thrombotic complications in critically ill ICU patients with COVID-19. Thromb Res 2020;191:145–7.

32. Jimenez D, Garcia-Sanchez A, Rali P, et al. Incidence of VTE and bleeding among hospitalized patients with Coronavirus disease 2019: a systematic review and meta-analysis. Chest 2021;159(3):1182–96.

33. Helms J, Tacquard C, Severac F, et al. High risk of thrombosis in patients with severe SARS-CoV-2 infection: a multicenter prospective cohort study. Intensive Care Med 2020;46(6):1089–98.

34. Barry O de, Mekki A, Diffre C, et al. Arterial and venous abdominal thrombosis in a 79-year-old woman with COVID-19 pneumonia. Radiol Case Rep 2020;15(7):1054–7.

35. Shah A, Donovan K, McHugh A, et al. Thrombotic and haemorrhagic complications in critically ill patients with COVID-19: a multicentre observational study. Crit Care 2020;24(1):561.

36. Oxley TJ, Mocco J, Majidi S, et al. Large-vessel stroke as a presenting feature of Covid-19 in the young. N Engl J Med 2020;382(20):e60.

37. Choudry FA, Hamshere SM, Rathod KS, et al. High thrombus burden in patients with COVID-19 presenting with ST-segment elevation myocardial infarction. J Am Coll Cardiol 2020;76(10):1168–76.

38. Bellosta R, Luzzani L, Natalini G, et al. Acute limb ischemia in patients with COVID-19 pneumonia. J Vasc Surg 2020;72(6):1864–72.

39. Merkler AE, Parikh NS, Mir S, et al. Risk of ischemic stroke in patients with Coronavirus disease 2019 (COVID-19) vs patients with influenza. JAMA Neurol 2020;77(11):1366–72. https://doi.org/10.1001/jamaneurol.2020.2730.

40. Qureshi AI, Baskett WI, Huang W, et al. Acute ischemic stroke and COVID-19. Stroke 2020;52(3):905–12.

41. Frankfurter C, Buchan TA, Kobulnik J, et al. Reduced rate of hospital presentations for heart failure during the Covid-19 pandemic in Toronto, Canada. Can J Cardiol 2020;36(10):1680–4.

42. Cox ZL, Lai P, Lindenfeld J. Decreases in acute heart failure hospitalizations during COVID-19. Eur J Heart Fail 2020;22(6):1045–6.

43. Petrilli CM, Jones SA, Yang J, et al. Factors associated with hospital admission and critical illness among 5279 people with coronavirus disease 2019 in New York City: prospective cohort study. BMJ 2020;369:m1966.

44. Alvarez-Garcia J, Lee S, Gupta A, et al. Prognostic impact of prior heart failure in patients hospitalized with COVID-19. J Am Coll Cardiol 2020;76(20):2334–48.

45. Yonas E, Alwi I, Pranata R, et al. Effect of heart failure on the outcome of COVID-19 — a meta analysis and

systematic review. Am J Emerg Med 2021;46: 204–11.

46. Kindermann I, Barth C, Mahfoud F, et al. Update on myocarditis. J Am Coll Cardiol 2012;59(9):779–92.

47. Kumar K, Guirgis M, Zieroth S, et al. Influenza myocarditis and myositis: case presentation and review of the literature. Can J Cardiol 2011;27(4): 514–22.

48. Alhogbani T. Acute myocarditis associated with novel Middle East respiratory syndrome coronavirus. Ann Saudi Med 2016;36(1):78–80.

49. Maisch B, Ristić AD, Hufnagel G, et al. Pathophysiology of viral myocarditis the role of humoral immune response. Cardiovasc Pathol 2002;11(2): 112–22.

50. Kawakami R, Sakamoto A, Kawai K, et al. Pathological evidence for SARS-CoV-2 as a cause of myocarditis. J Am Coll Cardiol 2021;77(3):314–25.

51. Rathore SS, Rojas GA, Sondhi M, et al. Myocarditis associated with Covid-19 disease: a systematic review of published case reports and case series. Int J Clin Pract 2021;75(11):e14470.

52. Boehmer TK, Kompaniyets L, Lavery AM, et al. Association between COVID-19 and myocarditis using hospital-based administrative data - United States, March 2020-January 2021. MMWR Morb Mortal Wkly Rep 2021;70(35):1228–32.

53. Sawalha K, Abozenah M, Kadado AJ, et al. Systematic review of COVID-19 related myocarditis: insights on management and outcome. Cardiovasc Revasc Med 2021;23:107–13.

54. Mele D, Flamigni F, Rapezzi C, et al. Myocarditis in COVID-19 patients: current problems. Intern Emerg Med 2021;16(5):1123–9.

55. Shah RM, Shah M, Shah S, et al. Takotsubo syndrome and COVID-19: associations and implications. Curr Probl Cardiol 2021;46(3):100763.

56. Moady G, Atar S. Stress-induced cardiomyopathy—considerations for diagnosis and management during the COVID-19 pandemic. Medicina 2022;58(2): 192.

57. Liu K, Fang YY, Deng Y, et al. Clinical characteristics of novel coronavirus cases in tertiary hospitals in Hubei Province. Chin Med J (Engl) 2020;133(9): 1025–31.

58. Cho JH, Namazi A, Shelton R, et al. Cardiac arrhythmias in hospitalized patients with COVID-19: a prospective observational study in the western United States. PLoS One 2020;15(12): e0244533.

59. Bhatla A, Mayer MM, Adusumalli S, et al. COVID-19 and cardiac arrhythmias. Heart Rhythm 2020;17(9): 1439–44.

60. DeLago AJ, Essa M, Ghajar A, et al. Incidence and mortality trends of atrial fibrillation/atrial flutter in the United States 1990 to 2017. Am J Cardiol 2021;148: 78–83.

61. Chen MY, Xiao FP, Kuai L, et al. Outcomes of atrial fibrillation in patients with COVID-19 pneumonia: a systematic review and meta-analysis. Am J Emerg Med 2021;50:661–9.

62. Harrison SL, Fazio-Eynullayeva E, Lane DA, et al. Atrial fibrillation and the risk of 30-day incident thromboembolic events, and mortality in adults $\geq$ 50 years with COVID-19. J Arrhythm 2020;37(1): 231–7.

63. Li Z, Shao W, Zhang J, et al. Prevalence of atrial fibrillation and associated mortality among hospitalized patients with COVID-19: a systematic review and meta-analysis. Front Cardiovasc Med 2021;8: 720129.

64. Louis D, Kennedy K, Saad M, et al. Pre-admission oral anticoagulation is associated with fewer thrombotic comlpications in patients admitted with COVID-19. J Am Coll Cardiol 2022;79(9S): 1798.

65. Rosenberg ES, Dufort EM, Udo T, et al. Association of Treatment with hydroxychloroquine or azithromycin with in-hospital mortality in patients with COVID-19 in New York State. JAMA 2020;323(24): 2493–502.

66. Cavalcanti AB, Zampieri FG, Rosa RG, et al. Hydroxychloroquine with or without azithromycin in mild-to-moderate covid-19. N Engl J Med 2020;383(21): 2041–52.

67. Patel YR, Louis DW, Atalay M, et al. Cardiovascular magnetic resonance findings in young adult patients with acute myocarditis following mRNA COVID-19 vaccination: a case series. J Cardiovasc Magn Reson 2021;23(1):101.

68. Shaw KE, Cavalcante JL, Han BK, et al. Possible association between COVID-19 vaccine and myocarditis: clinical and CMR findings. JACC Cardiovasc Imaging 2021;14(9):1856–61.

69. Witberg G, Barda N, Hoss S, et al. Myocarditis after Covid-19 vaccination in a large health care organization. N Engl J Med 2021;385(23).

70. Oster ME, Shay DK, Su JR, et al. Myocarditis cases reported after mRNA-based COVID-19 vaccination in the US from December 2020 to August 2021. JAMA 2022;327(4):331–40.

71. Kammen MS van, Sousa DA de, Poli S, et al. Characteristics and outcomes of patients with cerebral venous sinus thrombosis in SARS-CoV-2 vaccine-induced immune thrombotic thrombocytopenia. JAMA Neurol 2021;78(11):1314–23.

72. Cari L, Alhosseini MN, Fiore P, et al. Cardiovascular, neurological, and pulmonary events following vaccination with the BNT162b2, ChAdOx1 nCoV-19, and Ad26.COV2.S vaccines: an analysis of European data. J Autoimmun 2021;125: 102742.

73. Patone M, Mei XW, Handunnetthi L, et al. Risks of myocarditis, pericarditis, and cardiac arrhythmias

associated with COVID-19 vaccination or SARS-CoV-2 infection. Nat Med 2021;1–13. https://doi.org/10.1038/s41591-021-01630-0.

74. Xie Y, Xu E, Bowe B, et al. Long-term cardiovascular outcomes of COVID-19. Nat Med 2022;1–8. https://doi.org/10.1038/s41591-022-01689-3.

75. Crook H, Raza S, Nowell J, et al. Long covid—mechanisms, risk factors, and management. BMJ 2021;374:n1648.

76. Leong DP, Banerjee A, Yusuf S. COVID-19 vaccination prioritization on the basis of cardiovascular risk factors and number needed to vaccinate to prevent death. Can J Cardiol 2021;37(7):1112–6.

Use and Prognostic Implications of Cardiac Troponin in COVID-19

Laura De Michieli, MD[a,b], Allan S. Jaffe, MD[a,c], Yader Sandoval, MD[a,*]

KEYWORDS

- COVID-19 • Cardiac troponin • High sensitivity cardiac troponin • Myocardial injury
- Risk stratification • Prognosis

KEY POINTS

- For patients with COVID-19 infection, myocardial injury is diagnosed when cardiac troponin (cTn) concentrations exceed the 99th percentile upper-reference limit.
- Although myocardial injury is common, cTn increases are usually modest and criteria for myocardial infarction (MI) are infrequently met.
- While both direct and indirect mechanisms of myocardial damage play a role in acute myocardial injury during COVID-19, chronic myocardial injury related to comorbidities is frequently present.
- Myocardial injury has adverse short-term prognostic implications, with more data needed on long-term outcomes. The magnitude of cTn increases is also prognostic.

INTRODUCTION

The coronavirus disease 2019 (COVID-19) pandemic caused by the SARS-CoV-2 infection continues to have a severe global impact. Since the earliest reports from China,[1–3] it has been clear that cardiac involvement is frequent in patients with COVID-19, especially in those with concomitant cardiovascular comorbidities. The early studies had limitations due in part to arbitrary definitions for cardiac involvement.[4] Numerous studies have documented the value of cardiac troponin (cTn) to detect myocardial injury and for risk stratification. This review will discuss the latest information about cardiac involvement with an emphasis on the use of cTn.

DEFINITION OF MYOCARDIAL INJURY

Per the Fourth Universal Definition of Myocardial Infarction (4UDMI),[5] cTn is the biomarker of choice for the detection of myocardial injury and, in the proper clinical situation, the diagnosis of myocardial infarction (MI). If available, high-sensitivity (hs-cTn) cTn assays are preferred.[6] An assay is defined as high sensitivity if (a) the 99th percentile can be measured with analytical imprecision ≤10% and (b) the assay measures cTn concentrations above the limit of detection (LOD) in ≥50% of both healthy men and women.[7]

Myocardial injury is defined as any cTn increase above the assay-specific 99th percentile upper reference limit (URL) of a healthy population. When acute myocardial injury occurs, defined as a dynamic rising and/or falling pattern of cTn concentrations with at least one cTn concentration above the 99th percentile, and there are signs and/or symptoms of acute myocardial ischemia, a diagnosis of MI is made. Due to the increased sensitivity of hs-cTn assays, myocardial injury is detected far more frequently in a variety of clinical situations not related to myocardial ischemia than in those with MI.[5] It is often challenging for

This article originally appeared in Cardiology Clinics, Volume 40, Issue 3, August 2022.

[a] Department of Cardiovascular Diseases, Mayo Clinic, 200 1st Street Southwest, Rochester, MN 55905, USA; [b] Department of Cardiac, Thoracic, Vascular Sciences and Public Health, University of Padova, Via Giustiniani 2, Padova 35128, Italy; [c] Department of Laboratory Medicine and Pathology, Mayo Clinic, 200 1st Street Southwest, Rochester, MN 55905, USA

* Corresponding author.

E-mail address: sandoval.yader@mayo.edu

Heart Failure Clin 19 (2023) 163–176
https://doi.org/10.1016/j.hfc.2022.08.005

clinicians to identify the specific reason for hs-cTn elevations, as it can often occur in the critically ill. COVID-19 infections can induce alterations in myocardial oxygen consumption and contribute to ischemia but are also associated with pulmonary embolism (PE), critical illness, myocarditis, as well as the direct effects of SARS-CoV-2 on the myocardium and perhaps the microvasculature, making it challenging for clinicians to determine a discrete etiology.

ETIOLOGIES MYOCARDIAL INJURY IN COVID-19

There are multiple mechanisms that link COVID-19 disease to myocardial injury but also with other forms of cardiac involvement like heart failure (HF) with reduced ejection fraction and arrhythmias.[8] While clinicians often associate cTn increases in COVID-19 to direct effects, many patients often have clear antecedent causes for chronic injury like chronic cardiovascular disease that explain such elevations. In this section, we will analyze potential mechanisms of cardiac involvement that can lead to myocardial injury in this setting.

Direct Damage of SARS-CoV-2 in the Cardiovascular System

One possible mechanism for direct damage is the cytotoxic effect of SARS-CoV-2 on the endothelium which can cause diffuse microthrombosis.[9,10] At postmortem evaluation, nonocclusive fibrin microthrombi (without ischemic injury) are common (12/15 patients with COVID-19).[11]

Another potential mechanism is direct virus-induced myocardial injury and the potential for myocarditis. SARS-CoV-2 has been detected in the myocardium[12] and, in a multicenter autopsy study,[13] increased interstitial myocardial macrophages were identified in most of the cases but lymphocytic myocarditis in only a small fraction. Clinical studies suggest that myocarditis caused by SARS-CoV-2 is uncommon.[14]

Other hypotheses for direct damage include the possibility of infection and replication of virus within noncontractile cells in the heart such as endothelial cells, fibroblasts, and pericytes with matrix inflammation and fibrosis. There also are other speculative hypotheses.[9]

Nondirect Effects of SARS-CoV-2 in the Cardiovascular System

Nondirect effects of SARS-CoV-2 could be related to angiotensin-converting enzyme 2 (ACE2) downregulation/shedding with a subsequent hyperactive renin–angiotensin–aldosterone system (RAAS). Moreover, SARS-CoV-2 infection induces the activation of the innate immune system, leading to elevated levels of proinflammatory cytokines, including interleukin-6 (IL-6), interleukin-1, interleukin-2, tumor necrosis factor alpha, and interferon-c.[9]

Furthermore, SARS-CoV-2 can activate a cascade of thrombotic mechanisms through hyperactivated monocytes, platelets, and neutrophils generating neutrophil extracellular traps (NETs).[9] Indeed, hypercoagulation with diffuse microthrombi is considered the main cause of organ failure in severe cases.[11,13]

Viral Load and Myocardial Injury

There may be a relationship between viral load and myocardial injury. In one study,[15] all patients with detectable SARS-CoV-2 viral load had quantifiable ($\geq$6 ng/L) hs-cTnT concentrations, and 76% of them had concentrations above the assay-specific 99th percentile indicative of myocardial injury. While those without viremia also had quantifiable hs-cTnT concentrations (59% of cases) and myocardial injury (38%),[15] these abnormalities were significantly more common in those with viremia. Another report[16] evaluating both groups, however, concluded that there was no significant difference in the incidence of myocardial injury in patients with low compared with elevated viral load. Nonetheless, both myocardial injury and an elevated viral load were independent predictors of in-hospital mortality.[16] Finally, a study of symptomatic hospitalized patients suggest that patients with COVID-19 and viremia have higher concentrations of inflammatory markers (such as IL-6, C-reactive protein, procalcitonin, and ferritin), but similar levels of cTnT and NT-proBNP to patients without viremia.[17]

CLASSIFICATION OF MYOCARDIAL INJURY IN COVID-19

As suggested previously,[4] each cTn increase greater than the 99th percentile URL should be classified as chronic myocardial injury, acute nonischemic myocardial injury, or acute MI. **Fig. 1** summarizes this classification and some of the possible mechanisms of myocardial injury in patients with COVID-19.

Chronic Myocardial Injury

Chronic myocardial injury is defined as stable increases (<20% variation) above the 99th percentile of cTn concentrations.[5] Patients with COVID-19 are frequently affected by chronic

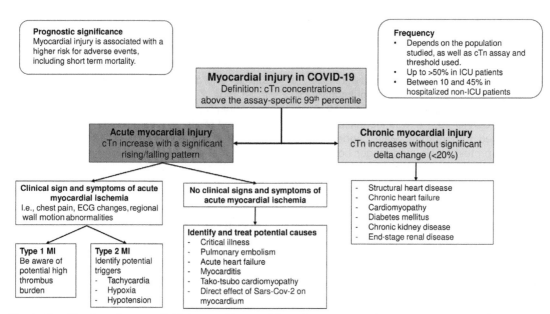

Fig. 1. Classification of myocardial injury and its possible pathogenetic mechanisms in patients with COVID-19.

cardiovascular comorbidities, such as hypertension, diabetes, coronary artery disease, HF, and chronic kidney disease (CKD),[1,3,18] all of which can be associated with cTn increases above the 99th percentile. Structural heart disease and HF are often associated with chronic cTn increases which portend an adverse prognosis.[5,19–21] Similarly, an elevated cTn in patients with diabetes and CKD identifies patients at higher risk of cardiovascular events.[22,23]

Studies in patients with COVID-19 with serial cTn measurements indicate that from 13% to 26% have stable and thus chronic increases in cTn.[24–26] In our multicenter Mayo Clinic health system study,[27] we adjudicated every hs-cTnT increase above the sex-specific 99th percentile among patients with COVID-19. Most hs-cTnT elevations were modest, with a median value of 12 ng/L, and significantly higher in men than in women (15 vs 9 ng/L). About half of the increases were associated with conditions such as HF, cardiomyopathy, or CKD. These data support the hypothesis that, in significant proportions of patients with COVID-19, myocardial injury is chronic and not due to effects directly related to COVID-19.

Acute Nonischemic Myocardial Injury

Acute nonischemic myocardial injury is defined as a significant rise and/or fall in cTn concentrations with at least one cTn concentration above the 99th percentile without clinical signs and symptoms of acute myocardial ischemia.[5] These occur often in critically ill patients[4,8] and are not specific to COVID-19. A recent study[28] comparing COVID-19 with influenza patients showed that, despite a higher absolute risk of death in patients with COVID-19, myocardial injury was frequent and increased the risk of death in both diseases. Moreover, acute myocardial injury is common in critically ill patients,[29] in those with acute respiratory distress,[30] and sepsis.[31] In our COVID-19 study,[27] we found that critical illness and sepsis could be identified as drivers of cTn increases in about 40% of patients. Metkus and colleagues[32] compared the frequency of myocardial injury in intubated patients with COVID-19 with patients with other causes of acute respiratory distress syndrome (ARDS) and reported that the rate of myocardial injury was similar (51% in COVID-19 compared with 49.6% in ARDS). They concluded that myocardial injury in severe COVID-19 is related to baseline comorbidities, advanced age, and multisystem organ dysfunction, like what happens in traditional ARDS. In addition to the multiorgan dysfunction and hemodynamic impairment that can lead to cTn increases, patients with severe sepsis and septic shock may manifest abnormal systolic function and impaired myocardial relaxation.[33] An echocardiography study in patients with COVID-19 reported that those with myocardial injury more frequently manifested left ventricular (LV) dysfunction detected by global longitudinal strain (GLS) and right ventricular (RV) dysfunction, which only partially resolved during follow-up.[34] Similarly, another study reported that patients with myocardial injury more frequently manifest global LV dysfunction, regional wall motion abnormalities, diastolic dysfunction, RV dysfunction, and pericardial effusions.[35]

Other causes of acute nonischemic myocardial injury include RV pressure overload related to PE[36,37] and/or microthrombi in the pulmonary circulation.[13] In a retrospective study[37] of 1240 patients with COVID-19, PE was identified in 8.3% by computed tomography. Male gender, higher C-reactive protein levels, and longer hospitalization were associated with higher risk of PE while anticoagulation (both at prophylactic and therapeutic dose) were protective. A meta-analysis[36] of 7178 patients with COVID-19 reported a pooled incidence of acute PE in 15% of patients hospitalized in general wards and in 23% of ICU patients.

Data on endomyocardial biopsy (EMB)/autopsy tissue characterization in suspected COVID-19 are scarce[38] but myocardial inflammation (without necrosis) caused by macrophages and T cells is common in noninfectious and in COVID-19 related deaths but usually without histologic criteria for myocarditis.[39] There are, however, a few cases of EMB/autopsy-proven histologic and immuno-histological active myocarditis but only 3 tested positive for SARS-CoV-2 by polymerase chain reaction on heart tissue suggesting the hypothesis that a virus-negative form, possibly triggered by the infection, might be etiologic.[38] In our report,[27] myocarditis was rare. There was clinical suspicion in 3 patients, but none had confirmatory testing performed.

Finally, features compatible with Takotsubo cardiomyopathy have been identified in 2% to 4%[40,41] of patients with COVID-19 undergoing transthoracic echocardiogram. It could develop from catecholamine-induced microvascular dysfunction or secondary to the metabolic, inflammatory, and emotional impairment associated with COVID-19.[41]

Type 1 and type 2 Myocardial Infarction

When reports demonstrated a high incidence of myocardial injury in patients with COVID-19, there were concerns about a possible high incidence of type 1 MI related to the prothrombotic state or, in those critically ill, type 2 MI. In our study[27] which used systematic adjudication[5] of all hs-cTnT increases, only a minority (5%) met MI criteria. Among those with type 2 MI, the most frequent triggers were hypoxia, hypotension, and/or tachyarrhythmias. Salbach and colleagues[26] reported a similarly low incidence. Differences in the frequency of type 2 MI in nonadjudicated studies are likely related to patient selection and less rigor in applying criteria establishing the presence of acute myocardial ischemia. One potential difference is that[42] in patients with COVID-19, oxygen demand-supply imbalance is often secondary to hypoxemia, increased heart rate, inflammatory status, and/or decompensated HF, whereas in most type 2 MIs, tachyarrhythmias and anemia are often prevalent mechanisms. Conventional treatment strategies seem appropriate but individualized care is warranted given the heterogeneous presentations and mechanisms. It is worth noting that in those with STEMI,[43] there seems to be a higher thrombus burden, and these patients can have worse outcomes.

FREQUENCY OF MYOCARDIAL INJURY IN PATIENTS WITH COVID-19

Many studies in this area have used arbitrary definitions and cutoffs to define myocardial injury[2,44] and others have been based on non-high sensitivity cTn assays.[45] **Table 1** tabulates the frequency of myocardial injury based on hs-cTn concentrations above the 99th percentile URL or above specified thresholds. As shown in **Fig. 2**, the frequency of myocardial injury varies widely probably in relation to patient selection. In studies of patients admitted to intensive care units (ICU), the frequency of myocardial injury is as high as or greater than 50%.[32,46,47] Studies that include a broader spectrum of patients suggest a frequency that ranges from 10%[48,49] to more than 45%.[26,27,50–52] This variation is likely related to the specific assay and/or threshold used, patient selection, and the population baseline characteristics. Only a small number of studies (see **Table 1**) applied sex-specific 99th percentiles as recommended.[5]

THE USE OF CARDIAC TROPONIN IN PATIENTS WITH COVID-19

Using high-sensitivity cTn assays, following guideline recommendations, sex-specific 99th percentile URLs should be used to define myocardial injury.[5] The use of uniform criteria will allow reporting in a comparable way between studies. Moreover, the prognostic significance of myocardial injury as defined by cTn concentrations greater than 99th percentile URL has been demonstrated repeatedly in the COVID-19 population. Irrespective of etiology, myocardial injury is associated with adverse events and increased mortality in patients with COVID-19.[2,45,51]

Single Sample Versus Serial Samples

Most studies only report values at baseline. Limited data exist addressing serial samples.

Table 1
Frequency of myocardial injury based on hs-cTn concentrations above the 99th percentile URL or above specified thresholds

Study	Location	Population	Cardiac Troponin Assay	Cutoffs Used	Frequency of Myocardial Injury
Cao et al,[63] 2020	Wuhan, China	244 COVID-19 admitted patients w/o CV disease or CKD	ADVIA Centaur XP, Siemens Healthcare Diagnostics, Erlangen, Germany).	>40 ng/L	11%
Li et al,[48] 2020	Wuhan, China	2068 COVID-19 admitted patients	Hs-cTnI, other details NR	>34.2 pg/mL	8.8% total, 2.3% in non-critically ill 30% in critically ill
Lorente-Ros et al,[64] 2020	Spain	707 COVID-19 admitted patients	Abbott hs-cTnI	> 14 ng/L	20.9%
Huang et al,[44] 2020	Wuhan, China.	41 COVID-19 admitted patients	Hs-cTnI, other details NR.	>28 ng/L	All: 12% ICU: 31% Non-ICU: 4%
Zhou F. et al,[3] 2020	Wuhan, China.	191 COVID-19 admitted patients	Hs-cTnI, other details NR	>28 pg/mL	All: 17% Non-survivor: 46% Survivor: 1%
Inciardi et al,[50] 2020	Brescia, Italy	99 COVID-19 admitted patients	Hs-TnT	>14 ng/L	71% of patients with cardiac disease, 47% without cardiac disease
Cecconi et al,[65] 2020	Milano, Italy	239 COVID-19 admitted patients	Troponin I, other details NR	>19.8 ng/L	27.7% overall
Nie et al,[66] 2020	Huazhong, China	311 COVID-19 admitted patients	hs-cTnI, ARCHITECT STAT, Abbott	>99th URL	33.1%
Wei et al,[67] 2020	China	101 COVID-19 admitted patients	hs-TnT	>14 ng/L	15.8%
Wang et al,[68] 2020	Wuhan, China	22 COVID-19 admitted patients with severe pneumonia	hs-cTnI, other details NR	>34.2 pg/mL	13%
Heberto et al,[69] 2020	Mexico	254 COVID-19 admitted patients	hs-cTnI Beckman Coulter	>17.5 ng/L	28.7%
Raad et al,[70] 2020	Southeast Michigan, USA	1020 COVID-19 admitted patients	hs-cTnI Beckman-Coulter	>18 ng/L	38%

(continued on next page)

Table 1
(continued)

Study	Location	Population	Cardiac Troponin Assay	Cutoffs Used	Frequency of Myocardial Injury
Stefanini et al,[71] 2020	Milan, Italy	397 COVID-19 admitted patients	hs-TnI Beckman Coulter	≥19.6 ng/L	25%
Schiavone et al,[72] 2020	Italy	674 COVID-19 admitted patients	Hs-cTn, other details NR	>99th URL	43.8% in CCS 14.4% without CCS
Arcari et al,[73] 2020	Rome, Italy	111 COVID-19 admitted patients	Hs-Troponin T Hs-Troponin I (other details NR)	< 14 pg/mL < 35 pg/mL	38%
Ghio et al,[74] 2020	Pavia, Italy	405 COVID-19 admitted patients	Hs-cTnI (other details NR)	99th URL	74/340 (22%)
Karbalai Saleh et al,[75] 2020	Tehran, Iran	386 COVID-19 admitted patients	hs-cTnI, other details NR	>26 ng/mL for men >11 ng/L for women	29.8%
Lombardi et al,[51] 2020	Italy, multicentric	614 COVID-19 patients admitted to Cardiology Units	Hs-cTnI or hs-cTnT, other details NR	>99th URL	45%
Salvatici et al,[76] 2020	Milan, Italy	523 COVID-19 admitted patients	hs-TnI Beckman Coulter	11.6 ng/L for women 19.8 ng/L for men	37.3%
Singh et al,[52] 2020	Chicago USA	276 COVID-19 admitted patients	Hs-TnT	17 ng/L (median in their population)	48%
Fan et al,[77] 2020	Wuhan china	353 COVID-19 admitted patients	Hs-cTnI STAT High Sensitive Troponin-I Abbott	>34.2 pg/mL for men >15.6 pg/mL for women	22.4%
He et al,[78] 2020	Wuhan china	1031 COVID-19 admitted patients	Hs-cTnI, other details NR	>99th URL	20.7%
Zaninotto el al.[24] 2020	Padova, Italy	113 COVID-19 admitted patients	Hs-cTnI Architect i2000, Abbott Diagnostics	16 ng/L for women 34 ng/L for men	45%
Ferrante et al,[79] 2020	Milano. Italy	332 COVID-19 admitted patients with chest CT	Hs-cTnI, other details NR	>20 ng/L	37%
Chen et al,[80] 2020	Wuhan china	726 COVID-19 admitted patients severe or critically ill	Hs-cTnI Architect i2000, Abbott Diagnostics	>28 ng/L	37.4% in critical patients 10.4% in severe patients
Poterucha et al,[81] 2021	New York, USA	887 COVID-19 admitted patients with ECG	Hs-cTnT	≥20 ng/L	43%

Study	Location	Population	Troponin	Assay	Cutoff	Prevalence
Perrone et al,[82] 2021	Italy, multicentric	543 COVID-19 admitted patients	hs-cTnT		>14 ng/L	47%
Metkus et al,[32] 2021	Baltimore, USA	243 COVID-19 admitted patients intubated.	Hs-cTnI and hs-cTnT		>99th URL	51%
Peiró et al,[83] 2021	Tarragona, Spain	196 COVID-19 patients ED/hospital	Hs-cTn I Assay, Advia Centaur, Siemens		>21 ng/L	39.3%
Efros et al,[84] 2021	Tel-Aviv, Israel	559 COVID-19 admitted patients	hs-TnT		>99th URL	28.4%
Cipriani et al,[85] 2021	Padova, Italy	109 COVID-19 admitted patients	Hs-cTnI Architect i2000, Abbott Diagnostics		16 ng/L for women 34 ng/L for men	38%
Qian et al,[86] 2021	Wuhan china	77 ICU COVID-19 patients	Hs-cTnI, other details NR		>28 ng/L	53%
De Michieli et al,[54] 2021	Padova, Italy	426 ED COVID-19 patients	Hs-cTnI Architect i2000, Abbott Diagnostics		16 ng/L for women 34 ng/L for men	27.2%
Siddiqi et al,[15] 2021	Boston, USA	70 COVID-19 admitted patients	Hs-cTnT		>14 ng/L	16/21 (76%) Pts with viremia 18/49 (38%) w/o viremia
Larcher et al,[47] 2021	France	111 ICU COVID-19 patients	Hs-cTnT		>14 ng/L	55%
Demir et al,[46] 2021	London, UK	176 ICU COVID-19 pts with cTn	Hs-cTnT		>14 ng/L	56%
Myhre et al,[17] 2021	Akershus University Hospital Norway	123 COVID-19 admitted patients	Hs-cTnT		>10 ng/L for women >15 ng/L for men	42% in pts with viremia 33% in pts w/o
Bieber et al,[34] 2021	Munich, Germany	32 COVID-19 admitted patients with 3D echo	Hs-cTnT		>14 ng/L	56%
Garcia de Guadiana-Romualdo et al,[87] 2021	Spain, multicenter	1280 ED COVID-19 patients	Hs-cTnT cTnI Siemens Atellica cTnI Siemens Advia Centaur cTn I Siemens Dimension EXL cTnI Abbott Architect cTn I Beckman Dxl 800/Access		>99th URL	26.9% w/o sex-specific cutoffs 30% with sex-specific cutoffs
de Falco et al,[49] 2021	Naples, Italy	174 COVID-19 admitted patients	Hs-cTnI Architect i2000, Abbott Diagnostics		16 ng/L for women 34 ng/L for men	11.5%
Barman et al,[58] 2021	Turkey	607 COVID-19 admitted patients	Hs-cTnI, other details NR		>14 pg/mL	24.7%
De Michieli et al,[27] 2021	USA, multicenter	367 COVID-19 admitted patients with cTn measured	Hs-cTnT		>10 ng/L for women, >15 ng/L for men	46%

(continued on next page)

Table 1
(continued)

Study	Location	Population	Cardiac Troponin Assay	Cutoffs Used	Frequency of Myocardial Injury
Ozer et al,[88] 2021	Turkey	73 COVID-19 admitted patients with Chest CT	Abbott, ARCHITECT STAT High Sensitive Troponin-I	>11.5 ng/L	39.7%
Caro-Codón et al,[89] 2021	Madrid, Spain	918 patients with COVID-19 ED with cTn measured	Atellica Solution IM1600, Siemens Healthineers hs-cTnI	> 34.1 ng/L > 53.5 ng/L	20.7%
Maino et al,[90] 2021	Rome, Italy	189 COVID-19 admitted patients	hs-TnI Advia Centaur Siemens	57 ng/L For men 37 ng/L for women	16% overall 9.7% in mild 29.0% in severe 61.3% in critical
Chehab et al,[16] 2021	Detroit, USA	270 COVID-19 admitted patients with cTn	Hs-cTnI Beckman Coulter	100 ng/L (not URL)	32.6%
Arcari et al,[91] 2021	Italy, multicenter	252 COVID-19 admitted patients, 229 with cTn	Hs-Troponin T hs-Troponin I, other details NR	14 pg/mL 35 pg/mL	36%
Salbach et al,[26] 2021	Heildeberg, Germany	104 COVID-19 admitted patients	Hs-cTnT	>14 ng/L	44.2%

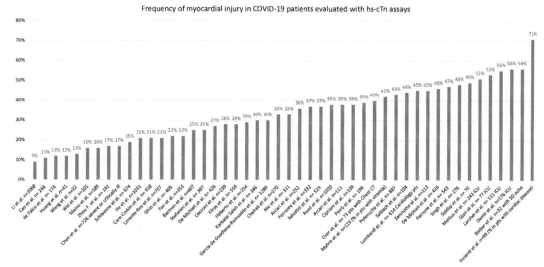

Fig. 2. Frequency of myocardial injury in multiple studies based on hs-cTn values. Details about different studies' population, the assays used, and a complete list of references are available on **Table 1**.

Kini and colleagues[25] evaluated hs-cTnI measurements between 72h before and 48h after the COVID19 diagnosis and classified patients as suffering from chronic myocardial injury or acute myocardial injury (>20% or >50% delta with elevated or normal baseline cTn, respectively). They found that both types of myocardial injury were associated with increased mortality at 30 days and 6 months even after multivariable adjustment. However, among patients less than 65 years and those without known coronary artery disease, acute myocardial injury was associated with a worse prognosis at 6 months. It was associated with a more pronounced inflammatory status, more ischemic risk factors such as intracoronary thrombosis and more oxygen supply–demand imbalance due to sepsis, but also more nonischemic conditions, like myocarditis, PE, and Takotsubo syndrome. In contrast, patients with chronic myocardial injury had more chronic comorbidities, including CKD and HF. Nuzzi and colleagues[53] evaluated hs-cTn measurements (either T or I) within 24 h of admission and, subsequently, again between 24 and 48 h. They categorized patients in 4 groups: normal (troponin <99th URL at both assessments), normal-elevated (normal cTn at admission and elevated thereafter), elevated-normal or elevated (ie, cTn>99th URL at both measurements). Patients with incident myocardial injury, with persistent elevated cTn, and with elevated cTn only at admission had a higher risk of death compared with those with normal cTn at both evaluations. By multivariable analysis, patients that developed myocardial injury

had the highest mortality risk. A smaller study[24] showed that patients with significant variation in concentrations of hs-cTnI (delta ≥ 20%), and at least one value ≥ 99th sex-specific URLs had longer hospital stays, more aggressive disease, and more often needed admission to ICU. Therefore, the data seem to indicate an adjunctive prognostic role for serial sampling although the populations that benefit most from this monitoring are a matter of debate.

Adjunctive Role of Cardiac Troponin in Risk Stratification

The role of very low hs-cTn concentrations to facilitate the identification of low-risk patients with a favorable prognosis has been demonstrated for both hs-cTnT[27] and hs-cTnI.[54] Patients with very low values at presentation (<6 ng/L for Roche hs-cTnT and < 5 ng/L for Abbott hs-cTnI) are at low risk for mortality and adverse events. Particularly, a single hs-cTnT less than 6 ng/L identified 26% of patients with COVID-19 without mortality and a low risk of major adverse events among patients presenting to the ED.[27] Similarly, an initial hs-cTnI *less than* 5 ng/L identified 33% of patients at low risk with 97.8% sensitivity and 99.2% negative predictive value in a hospitalized cohort.[54] These findings are similar to what is suggested for ruling-out MI, and likely occur because very low hs-cTn concentrations represent an objective measure to identify younger patients with fewer comorbidities.

Conversely, whether cTn increases enhance risk stratification in patients with COVID-19 remains a matter of debate. Omland and colleagues[55] reported that in multivariable models adjusting for clinical variables and a severity of illness score, only ferritin and lactate dehydrogenase (but not cTn) were significant predictors of a composite outcome of hospital mortality and admission to the ICU for mechanical ventilation and lasting greater than 24 hours in consecutive unselected COVID-19 patients. In our Padova study,[54] in patients with COVID-19 presenting through the ED, hs-cTnI was a significant predictor of mortality for patients with lower Acute Physiology and Chronic Health Evaluation II (APACHE II) score but not in those with higher (>13) APACE score. One could argue that in those that are more critically ill, the adjunctive role of cTn in predicting outcomes is more limited. However, hs-cTn can help to identify those who are less severely ill but are also at risk. Moreover, its use may be more clinically convenient than a more complex multivariable model. It may also be the case that many studies were based on cTn concentrations obtained for clinical reasons, potentially biasing the analysis.

When to Measure Cardiac Troponin and What to Do if It Is Elevated?

The European Society of Cardiology Study Group on Biomarkers in Cardiology of the Acute Cardiovascular Care Association developed a document discussing the significance and the proper use of cTn in COVID-19.[56] There is a paucity of evidence regarding the appropriate response to finding an increased hs-cTn concentration. If a type 1 MI is suspected, established diagnostic algorithms for rule-out and/or rule-in of MI should be deployed according to current guidelines.[56] However, given that in most patients with COVID-19 a type 1 MI is not present, these individuals rarely undergo coronary angiography. Indeed, in critically ill patients with septic shock and/or ARDS, cTn increases are more likely due to critical illness with or without hemodynamic impairment, resulting in myocardial injury or, if ischemia is present, type 2 MI.[56] Data on the appropriate therapy for type 2 MI in the critically ill are scarce and this is even more true for patients with COVID-19, constituting an important research gap.[57]

PROGNOSTIC IMPLICATIONS

Most studies have correlated myocardial injury with a poor in hospital outcome and short term mortality, regardless of the presence of known concomitant cardiovascular disease.[58,59] Conversely, cTn concentrations remain within the normal range in most survivors.[56] The incidence of myocardial injury increases with greater severity of illness and with the development of ARDS.[56] Regarding the consequences of myocardial injury in COVID-19, Kotecha and colleagues[60] performed cardiac magnetic resonance (CMR) in 148 patients with such injury who recovered from severe COVID-19 after a median of 68 days. They found late gadolinium enhancement and/or ischemia in 54% of patients. This included myocarditis-like scar in 26%, infarction and/or ischemia in 22%, and dual pathology in 6%. Myocarditis-like injury was limited in extent and had minimal functional consequences; however, in 30% signs of active myocarditis persisted. Of the patients with an ischemic injury pattern, 66% had no history of coronary disease suggesting pre-existing silent disease or de novo COVID-19-related changes. Puntmann and colleagues[61] performed CMR after a median of 71 days in 100 recovered patients with COVID-19 (including two-thirds of patients that recovered at home). hs-TnT was detectable in 71 patients and elevated (>13.9 pg/mL) in 5 patients. CMR revealed cardiac involvement in 78 patients and ongoing myocardial inflammation in 60. Hs-cTnT was significantly correlated with native T1 mapping, native T2 mapping, and LV mass.

Data regarding long-term consequences of myocardial injury in those who survived COVID-19 are scarce. A prospective exercise echocardiographic evaluation of 48 patients 6 months after COVID-19 disease (some of whom had experienced myocardial injury[62]) revealed that exercise induced a significant increase in the average E/e′ ratio and systolic pulmonary artery pressure in those who had suffered myocardial injury.

SUMMARY

Myocardial injury, defined as cTn increases above the assay-specific 99th percentile, is frequent in patients with COVID-19. It correlates with adverse events and short-term mortality. Most increases seem related to chronic cardiovascular conditions and acute nonischemic myocardial injury, similarly to that reported in severely ill patients. However, some studies with advanced cardiac imaging and long-term follow-up indicate that myocardial injury might be associated with long-term structural abnormalities and worse cardiac performance. Except for patients suffering from type 1 MI, the appropriate treatment of patients with COVID-19 with myocardial injury remains case-specific and further investigations are necessary to understand how to improve outcomes in this population.

CLINICS CARE POINTS

- Myocardial injury is common in patients with COVID-19 infection, but its frequency varies widely based on the population studied and the cTn assay and threshold used.

- Even though COVID-19 patients can present with type 1 or type 2 MI, acute and chronic myocardial injury (cTn increases above the 99th percentile without clinical evidence of acute myocardial ischemia) are the most common reasons for cTn increases.

- Regardless of the mechanism, myocardial injury, and the magnitude of cTn increases have prognostic significance.

DISCLOSURE

Dr Y. Sandoval has previously served on the Advisory Boards for Roche Diagnostics and Abbott Diagnostics without personal compensation. He has also been a speaker without personal financial compensation for Abbott Diagnostics. Dr A.S. Jaffe has consulted or presently consults for most of the major diagnostics companies, including Beckman-Coulter, Abbott, Siemens, Ortho Diagnostics, ET Healthcare, Roche, Radiometer, Sphingotec, RCE, and Amgen and Novartis. Dr L. De Michieli has nothing to disclose.

REFERENCES

1. Guo T, Fan Y, Chen M, et al. Cardiovascular implications of Fatal outcomes of patients with coronavirus disease 2019 (COVID-19). JAMA Cardiol 2020; 5(7):811.
2. Shi S, Qin M, Shen B, et al. Association of cardiac injury with mortality in hospitalized patients with COVID-19 in Wuhan, China. JAMA Cardiol 2020;5: 802–10.
3. Zhou F, Yu T, Du R, et al. Clinical course and risk factors for mortality of adult inpatients with COVID-19 in Wuhan, China: a retrospective cohort study. Lancet 2020;395(10229):1054–62.
4. Sandoval Y, Januzzi JL, Jaffe AS. Cardiac troponin for assessment of myocardial injury in COVID-19. J Am Coll Cardiol 2020;76(10):1244–58.
5. Thygesen K, Alpert JS, Jaffe AS, et al. Fourth Universal definition of myocardial infarction (2018). Circulation 2018;138(20).
6. Sandoval Y, Jaffe AS. Using high-sensitivity cardiac troponin T for acute cardiac care. Am J Med 2017; 130(12):1358–65.e1.
7. Apple FS, Jaffe AS, Collinson P, et al. IFCC educational materials on selected analytical and clinical applications of high sensitivity cardiac troponin assays. Clin Biochem 2015;48(4–5):201–3.
8. Jaffe AS, Cleland JGF, Katus HA. Myocardial injury in severe COVID-19 infection. Eur Heart J 2020; 41(22):2080–2.
9. Pesce M, Agostoni P, Bøtker HE, et al. COVID-19-related cardiac complications from clinical evidences to basic mechanisms: opinion paper of the ESC Working Group on Cellular Biology of the Heart. Cardiovasc Res 2021;117(10):2148–60.
10. Libby P, Lüscher T. COVID-19 is, in the end, an endothelial disease. Eur Heart J 2020;41(32): 3038–44.
11. Bois MC, Boire NA, Layman AJ, et al. COVID-19–Associated Nonocclusive fibrin microthrombi in the heart. Circulation 2021;143(3):230–43.
12. Tavazzi G, Pellegrini C, Maurelli M, et al. Myocardial localization of coronavirus in COVID-19 cardiogenic shock. Eur J Heart Fail 2020;22(5):911–5.
13. Basso C, Leone O, Rizzo S, et al. Pathological features of COVID-19-associated myocardial injury: a multicentre cardiovascular pathology study. Eur Heart J 2020;41(39):3827–35.
14. Ozieranski K, Tyminska A, Jonik S, et al. Clinically suspected myocarditis in the course of severe acute respiratory syndrome novel coronavirus-2 infection: Fact or Fiction? J Card Fail 2021;27(1):92–6.
15. Siddiqi HK, Weber B, Zhou G, et al. Increased prevalence of myocardial injury in patients with SARS-CoV-2 viremia. Am J Med 2021;134(4):542–6.
16. Chehab O, El Zein S, Kanj A, et al. SARS-CoV-2 viral load and myocardial injury: independent and Incremental predictors of adverse outcome. Mayo Clinic Proc Innov Qual Outcomes 2021;5(5):891–7.
17. Myhre PL, Prebensen C, Jonassen CM, et al. SARS-CoV-2 viremia is associated with inflammatory, but not cardiovascular biomarkers, in patients hospitalized for COVID-19. JAHA 2021;10(9).
18. Wu C, Chen X, Cai Y, et al. Risk factors associated with acute respiratory distress syndrome and death in patients with coronavirus disease 2019 pneumonia in Wuhan, China. JAMA Intern Med 2020; 180(7):934.
19. de Lemos JA, Drazner MH, Omland T, et al. Association of troponin T detected with a highly sensitive assay and cardiac structure and mortality risk in the general population. JAMA 2010;304(22):2503.
20. Takashio S, Yamamuro M, Izumiya Y, et al. Coronary microvascular dysfunction and diastolic load correlate with cardiac troponin T Release measured by a highly sensitive assay in patients with nonischemic heart failure. J Am Coll Cardiol 2013;62(7):632–40.
21. Myhre PL, Claggett B, Ballantyne CM, et al. Association between Circulating troponin concentrations, left ventricular systolic and diastolic functions, and

incident heart failure in Older Adults. JAMA Cardiol 2019;4(10):997.

22. Dillmann WH. Diabetic cardiomyopathy: what is it and can it Be Fixed? Circ Res 2019;124(8):1160–2.

23. Patel PC, Ayers CR, Murphy SA, et al. Association of Cystatin C with left ventricular structure and function: the Dallas heart study. Circ Heart Fail 2009;2(2): 98–104.

24. Zaninotto M, Mion MM, Padoan A, et al. Cardiac troponin I in SARS-CoV-2-patients: the additional prognostic value of serial monitoring. Clin Chim Acta 2020;511:75–80.

25. Kini A, Cao D, Nardin M, et al. Types of myocardial injury and mid-term outcomes in patients with COVID-19. Eur Heart J - Qual Care Clin Outcomes 2021;7(5):438–46.

26. Salbach C, Mueller-Hennessen M, Biener M, et al. Interpretation of myocardial injury subtypes in COVID-19 disease per fourth version of Universal Definition of Myocardial Infarction. Biomarkers 2021;26(5):401–9.

27. De Michieli L, Ola O, Knott JD, et al. High-sensitivity cardiac troponin T for the detection of myocardial injury and risk stratification in COVID-19. Clin Chem 2021;67(8):1080–9.

28. Biasco L, Klersy C, Beretta GS, et al. In: Bäck M, editor. Comparative frequency and prognostic impact of myocardial injury in hospitalized patients with COVID-19 and Influenza. European heart Journal Open. 2021. oeab025.

29. Babuin L, Vasile VC, Rio Perez JA, et al. Elevated cardiac troponin is an independent risk factor for short- and long-term mortality in medical intensive care unit patients. Crit Care Med 2008;36(3):759–65.

30. Vasile VC, Chai HS, Khambatta S, et al. Significance of elevated cardiac troponin T levels in critically ill patients with acute respiratory disease. Am J Med 2010;123(11):1049–58.

31. Vasile VC, Chai HS, Abdeldayem D, et al. Elevated cardiac troponin T levels in critically ill patients with sepsis. Am J Med 2013;126(12):1114–21.

32. Metkus TS, Sokoll LJ, Barth AS, et al. Myocardial injury in severe COVID-19 compared with non–COVID-19 acute respiratory distress syndrome. Circulation 2021;143(6):553–65.

33. Landesberg G, Jaffe AS, Gilon D, et al. Troponin elevation in severe sepsis and septic shock: the role of left ventricular diastolic dysfunction and right ventricular Dilatation. Crit Care Med 2014;42(4): 790–800.

34. Bieber S, Kraechan A, Hellmuth JC, et al. Left and right ventricular dysfunction in patients with COVID-19-associated myocardial injury. Infection 2021;49(3):491–500.

35. Giustino G, Croft LB, Stefanini GG, et al. Characterization of myocardial injury in patients with COVID-19. J Am Coll Cardiol 2020;76(18):2043–55.

36. Roncon L, Zuin M, Barco S, et al. Incidence of acute pulmonary embolism in COVID-19 patients: systematic review and meta-analysis. Eur J Intern Med 2020;82:29–37.

37. Fauvel C, Weizman O, Trimaille A, et al. Pulmonary embolism in COVID-19 patients: a French multicentre cohort study. Eur Heart J 2020;41(32): 3058–68.

38. Caforio ALP, Baritussio A, Basso C, et al. Clinically suspected and biopsy-proven myocarditis Temporally associated with SARS-CoV-2 infection. Annu Rev Med 2022;73(1). annurev-med-042220-023859.

39. Kawakami R, Sakamoto A, Kawai K, et al. Pathological evidence for SARS-CoV-2 as a cause of myocarditis. J Am Coll Cardiol 2021;77(3): 314–25.

40. Dweck MR, Bularga A, Hahn RT, et al. Global evaluation of echocardiography in patients with COVID-19. Eur Heart J - Cardiovasc Imaging 2020;21(9):949–58.

41. Giustino G, Croft LB, Oates CP, et al. Takotsubo cardiomyopathy in COVID-19. J Am Coll Cardiol 2020; 76(5):628–9.

42. Talanas G, Dossi F, Parodi G. Type 2 myocardial infarction in patients with coronavirus disease 2019. J Cardiovasc Med (Hagerstown) 2021;22: 603–5.

43. Choudry FA, Hamshere SM, Rathod KS, et al. High thrombus burden in patients with COVID-19 presenting with ST-Segment elevation myocardial infarction. J Am Coll Cardiol 2020;76(10):1168–76.

44. Huang C, Wang Y, Li X, et al. Clinical features of patients infected with 2019 novel coronavirus in Wuhan, China. Lancet 2020;395(10223): 497–506.

45. Lala A, Johnson KW, Januzzi JL, et al. Prevalence and Impact of myocardial injury in patients hospitalized with COVID-19 infection. J Am Coll Cardiol 2020;76(5):533–46.

46. Demir OM, Ryan M, Cirillo C, et al. Impact and determinants of high-sensitivity cardiac troponin-T concentration in patients with COVID-19 admitted to critical care. Am J Cardiol 2021;147:129–36.

47. Larcher R, Besnard N, Akouz A, et al. Admission high-sensitive cardiac troponin T level increase is independently associated with higher mortality in critically ill patients with COVID-19: a multicenter study. JCM 2021;10(8):1656.

48. Li C, Jiang J, Wang F, et al. Longitudinal correlation of biomarkers of cardiac injury, inflammation, and coagulation to outcome in hospitalized COVID-19 patients. J Mol Cell Cardiol 2020;147:74–87.

49. de Falco R, Vargas M, Palma D, et al. B-type natriuretic peptides and high-sensitive troponin I as COVID-19 survival factors: which one is the best performer? JCM 2021;10(12):2726.

50. Inciardi RM, Adamo M, Lupi L, et al. Characteristics and outcomes of patients hospitalized for COVID-19

and cardiac disease in Northern Italy. Eur Heart J 2020;41(19):1821–9.

51. Lombardi CM, Carubelli V, Iorio A, et al. Association of troponin levels with mortality in Italian patients hospitalized with coronavirus disease 2019: Results of a multicenter study. JAMA Cardiol 2020;5(11): 1274.

52. Singh N, Anchan RK, Besser SA, et al. High sensitivity Troponin-T for prediction of adverse events in patients with COVID-19. Biomarkers 2020;25(8): 626–33.

53. Nuzzi V, Merlo M, Specchia C, et al. The prognostic value of serial troponin measurements in patients admitted for COVID-19. ESC Heart Fail 2021;8: 3504–11.

54. De Michieli L, Babuin L, Vigolo S, et al. Using high sensitivity cardiac troponin values in patients with SARS-CoV-2 infection (COVID-19): the Padova experience. Clin Biochem 2021;90:8–14.

55. Omland T, Prebensen C, Røysland R, et al. Established cardiovascular biomarkers Provide limited prognostic information in unselected patients hospitalized with COVID-19. Circulation 2020;142(19): 1878–80.

56. Mueller C, Giannitsis E, Jaffe AS, et al. Cardiovascular biomarkers in patients with COVID-19. Eur Heart J Acute Cardiovasc Care 2021;10(3):310–9.

57. Bularga A, Chapman AR, Mills NL. Mechanisms of myocardial injury in COVID-19. Clin Chem 2021; 67(8):1044–6.

58. Barman HA, Atici A, Sahin I, et al. Prognostic significance of cardiac injury in COVID-19 patients with and without coronary artery disease. Coron Artery Dis 2021;32(5):359–66.

59. Çınar T, Hayıroğlu Mİ, Çiçek V, et al. Prognostic significance of cardiac troponin level in Covid-19 patients without known cardiovascular risk factors. Am J Emerg Med 2021;45:595–7.

60. Kotecha T, Knight DS, Razvi Y, et al. Patterns of myocardial injury in recovered troponin-positive COVID-19 patients assessed by cardiovascular magnetic resonance. Eur Heart J 2021;42(19):1866-1878. doi:10.1093/eurheartj/ehab075.

61. Puntmann VO, Carerj ML, Wieters I, et al. Outcomes of cardiovascular magnetic resonance imaging in patients recently recovered from coronavirus disease 2019 (COVID-19). JAMA Cardiol 2020;5(11):1265.

62. Fayol A, Livrozet M, Boutouyrie P, et al. Cardiac performance in patients hospitalized with COVID-19: a 6 month follow-up study. ESC Heart Fail 2021;8(3): 2232–9.

63. Cao J, Zheng Y, Luo Z, et al. Myocardial injury and COVID-19: Serum hs-cTnI level in risk stratification and the prediction of 30-day fatality in COVID-19 patients with no prior cardiovascular disease. Theranostics 2020;10(21):9663–73. https://doi.org/10. 7150/thno.47980.

64. Lorente-Ros A, Ruiz JMM, Rincón LM, et al. Myocardial injury determination improves risk stratification and predicts mortality in COVID-19 patients. Cardiol J 2020;27(4):8.

65. Cecconi M, Piovani D, Brunetta E, et al. Early predictors of clinical Deterioration in a cohort of 239 patients hospitalized for Covid-19 infection in Lombardy. Italy JCM 2020;9(5):1548. https://doi. org/10.3390/jcm9051548.

66. Nie SF, Yu M, Xie T, et al. Cardiac troponin I is an independent predictor for mortality in hospitalized patients with coronavirus disease 2019. Circulation 2020;120: 048789. https://doi.org/10.1161/CIRCULATIONAHA. 120.048789.

67. Wei JF, Huang FY, Xiong TY, et al. Acute myocardial injury is common in patients with COVID-19 and impairs their prognosis. Heart 2020;106(15): 1154–9. https://doi.org/10.1136/heartjnl-2020-317007.

68. Wang Y, Zheng Y, Tong Q, et al. Cardiac injury and clinical course of patients with coronavirus disease 2019. Front Cardiovasc Med 2020;7:147. https:// doi.org/10.3389/fcvm.2020.00147.

69. Heberto AB, Carlos PCJ, Antonio CRJ, et al. Implications of myocardial injury in Mexican hospitalized patients with coronavirus disease 2019 (COVID-19). IJC Heart & Vasculature 2020;30:100638. https://doi.org/10.1016/j.ijcha.2020.100638.

70. Raad M, Dabbagh M, Gorgis S, et al. Cardiac injury patterns and Inpatient outcomes among patients admitted with COVID-19. Am J Cardiol 2020;133: 154–61. https://doi.org/10.1016/j.amjcard.2020.07. 040.

71. Stefanini GG, Chiarito M, Ferrante G, et al. Early detection of elevated cardiac biomarkers to optimise risk stratification in patients with COVID-19. Heart 2020;106(19):1512–8. https://doi.org/10.1136/ heartjnl-2020-317322.

72. Schiavone M, Gasperetti A, Mancone M, et al. Redefining the prognostic value of high-sensitivity troponin in COVID-19 patients: the importance of concomitant coronary artery disease. JCM 2020; 9(10):3263. https://doi.org/10.3390/jcm9103263.

73. Arcari L, Luciani M, Cacciotti L, et al. Incidence and determinants of high-sensitivity troponin and natriuretic peptides elevation at admission in hospitalized COVID-19 pneumonia patients. Intern Emerg Med 2020;15(8):1467–76. https://doi.org/10.1007/ s11739-020-02498-7.

74. Ghio S, Baldi E, Vicentini A, et al. Cardiac involvement at presentation in patients hospitalized with COVID-19 and their outcome in a tertiary referral hospital in Northern Italy. Intern Emerg Med 2020; 15(8):1457–65. https://doi.org/10.1007/s11739-020-02493-y.

75. Karbalai Saleh S, Oraii A, Soleimani A, et al. The association between cardiac injury and outcomes in

hospitalized patients with COVID-19. Intern Emerg Med 2020;15(8):1415–24. https://doi.org/10.1007/s11739-020-02466-1.

76. Salvatici M, Barbieri B, Cioffi SMG, et al. Association between cardiac troponin I and mortality in patients with COVID-19. Biomarkers 2020;25(8):634–40. https://doi.org/10.1080/1354750X.2020.1831609.

77. Fan Q, Zhu H, Zhao J, et al. Risk factors for myocardial injury in patients with coronavirus disease 2019 in China. ESC Heart Fail 2020;7(6):4108–17. https://doi.org/10.1002/ehf2.13022.

78. He X, Wang L, Wang H, et al. Factors associated with acute cardiac injury and their effects on mortality in patients with COVID-19. Sci Rep 2020;10(1):20452. https://doi.org/10.1038/s41598-020-77172-1.

79. Ferrante G, Fazzari F, Cozzi O, et al. Risk factors for myocardial injury and death in patients with COVID-19: insights from a cohort study with chest computed tomography. Cardiovasc Res 2020;116(14):2239–46. https://doi.org/10.1093/cvr/cvaa193.

80. Chen H, Li X, Marmar T, et al. Cardiac Troponin I association with critical illness and death risk in 726 seriously ill COVID-19 patients: a retrospective cohort study. Int J Med Sci 2021;18(6):1474–83. https://doi.org/10.7150/ijms.53641.

81. Poterucha TJ, Elias P, Jain SS, et al. Admission cardiac diagnostic testing with Electrocardiography and troponin measurement Prognosticates increased 30-day mortality in COVID-19. JAHA 2021;10(1). https://doi.org/10.1161/JAHA.120.018476.

82. Perrone MA, Spolaore F, Ammirabile M, et al. The assessment of high sensitivity cardiac troponin in patients with COVID-19: a multicenter study. IJC Heart & Vasculature 2021;32:100715. https://doi.org/10.1016/j.ijcha.2021.100715.

83. Peiró ÓM, Carrasquer A, Sánchez-Gimenez R, et al. Biomarkers and short-term prognosis in COVID-19. Biomarkers 2021;26(2):119–26. https://doi.org/10.1080/1354750X.2021.1874052.

84. Efros O, Barda N, Meisel E, et al. Myocardial injury in hospitalized patients with COVID-19 infection—risk factors and outcomes. In: Ai T, editor. PLoS ONE 2021;16(2):e0247800. https://doi.org/10.1371/journal.pone.0247800.

85. Cipriani A, Capone F, Donato F, et al. Cardiac injury and mortality in patients with Coronavirus disease 2019 (COVID-19): insights from a mediation analysis. Intern Emerg Med 2021;16(2):419–27. https://doi.org/10.1007/s11739-020-02495-w.

86. Qian H, Gao P, Tian R, et al. Myocardial injury on admission as a risk in critically ill COVID-19 patients: a retrospective in-ICU study. J Cardiothorac Vasc Anesth 2021;35(3):846–53. https://doi.org/10.1053/j.jvca.2020.10.019.

87. García de Guadiana-Romualdo L, Morell-García D, Rodríguez-Fraga O, et al. Cardiac troponin and COVID-19 severity: Results from BIOCOVID study. Eur J Clin Invest 2021;51(6). https://doi.org/10.1111/eci.13532.

88. Özer S, Bulut E, Özyıldız AG, et al. Myocardial injury in COVID-19 patients is associated with the thickness of epicardial adipose tissue. Kardiologiia 2021;61(8):48–53. https://doi.org/10.18087/cardio.2021.8.n1638.

89. Caro-Codón J, Rey JR, Buño A, et al. Characterization of myocardial injury in a cohort of patients with SARS-CoV-2 infection. Medicina Clínica 2021;157(6):274–80. https://doi.org/10.1016/j.medcli.2021.02.001.

90. Maino A, Di Stasio E, Grimaldi MC, et al. Prevalence and characteristics of myocardial injury during COVID-19 pandemic: a new role for high-sensitive troponin. Int J Cardiol 2021;338:278–85. https://doi.org/10.1016/j.ijcard.2021.06.028.

91. Arcari L, Luciani M, Cacciotti L, et al. Coronavirus disease 2019 in patients with cardiovascular disease: clinical features and implications on cardiac biomarkers assessment. J Cardiovasc Med 2021;22(11):832–9. https://doi.org/10.2459/JCM.0000000000001252.

Review of Immunologic Manifestations of COVID-19 Infection and Vaccination

Valeriya Pozdnyakova, BS[a], Brittany Weber, MD, PhD[b],
Susan Cheng, MD, MPH, MMSc[c], Joseph E. Ebinger, MD, MS[c],*

KEYWORDS

• COVID-19 • Vaccination • Infection • Humoral immunity • Cellular immunity • Cardiovascular

KEY POINTS

- The severity of COVID-19 illness is directly correlated with early humoral immune response and inversely related with early cellular immune response.
- Innate immune response in pulmonary tissue may be partially evaded by SARS-CoV-2.
- Humoral and cellular immune responses elicited by vaccination wane approximately 6 months after initial vaccination, particularly among men and those over the age of 65.
- An additional vaccine dose can enhance immune protection following waning initial vaccine protection.
- Dysregulated immune response is associated with the severity of COVID-19 disease, including the development of acute respiratory distress syndrome (ARDS) and organ-specific sequelae such as myocarditis.

SIGNIFICANCE

In March 2020 the World Health Organization declared coronavirus disease 2019 (COVID-19) a global pandemic. As of January 28, 2022, there have been 364 million confirmed cases of COVID-19 and 5.6 million deaths around the globe.[1] In addition to causing overwhelming amounts of human suffering, COVID-19 has devastated health care systems, economies, and the social structures of daily life. Understanding how the human immune system responds to and overcomes SARS-CoV-2 infection is paramount to the discovery of effective treatments and prevention of severe disease.

VIROLOGY OF SARS-CoV-2

Understanding the immunologic response to SARS-CoV-2 requires understanding the virus' structure, transmissibility, and fatality. SARS-CoV-2 is an enveloped virus with a single-stranded positive sense RNA genome.[2] Like most coronaviruses, SARS-CoV-2 has 4 structural proteins: the nucleocapsid (N) protein which forms a helical structure around the viral genomic RNA and the spike (S), membrane (M), and envelope (E) proteins that are embedded in the outer lipid bilayer.[2] Each of these structural factors plays an important role in the infectivity and immunogenicity of the virus. Phylogenic analysis of SARS-

This article originally appeared in Cardiology Clinics, Volume 40, Issue 3, August 2022.
Funded by: NIH/NHLBI Grant number(s): K23HL 153888-02.
[a] F. Widjaja Foundation Inflammatory Bowel and Immunobiology Research Institute, Cedars-Sinai Medical Center, 8700 Beverly Boulevard, D4005, Los Angeles, CA 90048, USA; [b] Carl J. and Ruth Shapiro Cardiovascular Center, Brigham and Women's Hospital, 70 Francis Street, Boston, MA 02115, USA; [c] Department of Cardiology, Smidt Heart Institute, Cedars-Sinai Medical Center, 127 South Vicente Boulevard, Suite A3100, Los Angeles, CA 90048, USA
* Corresponding author.
E-mail address: Joseph.Ebinger@csmc.edu

CoV-2 revealed it to be in the same subgenus as the severe acute respiratory syndrome (SARS) coronavirus (SARS-CoV) and several other bat coronaviruses.[3] Out of the 7 coronaviruses infecting humans, 3 are known to be capable of replicating in the lower respiratory tract and causing severe disease: SARS-CoV, SARS-CoV-2, and Middle East respiratory syndrome coronavirus (MERS-CoV).[4]

The 2003 SARS and 2012 MERS outbreaks had case fatality rates of 10% and 34%, respectively, while most of the COVID-19 cases have remained relatively mild in comparison.[4] Specifically, the reported case fatality rate of COVID-19 peaked at 7.2% in April of 2020, declining to 2.2% by December 2020.[5] In the context of its lower mortality rate, SARS-CoV-2 is substantially more contagious than SARS-CoV and MERS-CoV.[6–8] This remarkable transmissibility, paired with its lower case fatality rate, has served as a double-edged sword given that milder illness affecting most of the cases has hampered public compliance with masking and social distancing recommendations.[9,10]

SARS-CoV-2 is spread through respiratory droplets and binds to the angiotensin-converting enzyme 2 (ACE2) receptor in nasal and bronchial epithelial cells and pneumocytes via viral S-protein.[11,12] The S-protein has 2 subunits, S1 and S2; S1 mediates binding to the host cell ACE2 receptor through the receptor-binding domain (RBD) while S2 directs viral cell membrane fusion. By comparison, the RBD of SARS-CoV-2 binds ACE2 with 5 to 10 times greater affinity than the RBD of SARS-CoV.[6,7] The recognition of the S-protein's importance in the cellular entry has made it a key target for the immune response, as well as vaccine-mediated protection.

IMMUNE RESPONSES TO SARS-CoV-2 INFECTION
Innate Immune Response in the Respiratory Tract

Human expression of ACE2 occurs on epithelial cells in both the upper and lower respiratory tract, with nasal epithelial cells expressing slightly greater amounts, making it an ideal environment for SARS-CoV-2 to enter the body.[13] As such, early immune activation often begins in these locations. A study of *ex vivo* SARS-CoV-2 infected turbinate tissue identified a broad and robust innate immune response in nasal tissue, with increased upregulation of interferon-stimulated genes (ISGs) and cytokine release, vital components in inhibiting viral infection of nucleated cells.[13,14] Comparatively, this response to SARS-CoV-2 was larger than that initiated by the influenza virus, characterized by significant upregulation of genes that specifically enhanced antigen presentation and immune cell signaling, indicating a robust immune recognition and response to the virus in the nose. SARS-CoV-2 infected lung tissue, on the other hand, failed to upregulate INF types I, II, and III. Upregulation of ISGs in infected lung tissue was observed, but cellular immune pathways such as antigen presentation, immune cell maturation, TNF receptor signaling, and inflammasome pathways were not activated.[13] In effect, an early innate immune response is initiated in both the upper and lower respiratory tracts; however, the downstream effect is blunted in the pulmonary tissue.

A possible explanation for this finding is the action of SARS-CoV-2 nonstructural protein 1 (NSP1) which inactivates the translational activity of the human 40S ribosomal subunit, a key link in the chain in the activation of the immune response following antigen detection.[8,15] Failure to translate the upregulation of ISGs could potentially explain the restricted innate response observed in the lung tissue. How nasal, but not lung, epithelial tissue overcomes the translation inhibiting effects of NSP1 is not yet understood. Other studies support this finding, demonstrating that in vitro SARS-CoV-2 infected primary human airway epithelial cultures are unable to produce type I or III IFN, yet the addition of exogenous IFN was able to significantly reduce viral burden in the same cultures.[16] This suggests that the SARS-CoV-2 inhibition of IFN production, not reduced susceptibility to INF's antiviral inducing mechanisms, may play an important role in the virus's ability to modulate and evade the immune response.

Immune Response and Severity of Illness

Growing evidence links the type and temper of the host immune response to SARS-CoV-2 infection with the severity of illness experienced by those infected.[17,18] A study by Almendro-Vasquez et al. compared the humoral and cellular responses to COVID-19 infection among patients who experienced a range of symptoms from mild to severe, both in the acute setting, as well as 4 to 7 months following recovery.[18] Patients with mild infection were well enough to convalesce at home and experienced minimal symptoms, while those with moderate disease were hospitalized, required oxygen, or had nonsevere acute respiratory distress syndrome (ARDS). Comparatively, severe infection was characterized by admission to the ICU, a P:F ratio of less than 200, or death from COVID-19. The researchers found that among patients with mild disease, the development of anti-S1 IgG antibodies was delayed nearly 2 weeks from symptom onset and that once formed, these antibodies demonstrated only modest neutralizing capacity.[18] Most patients in the moderate cohort also lacked detectable anti-S1 IgG for several weeks following symptom onset, however, once present, antibody levels were higher and consistent with robust neutralizing capacity. Comparatively, patients with severe illness had detectable anti-S1 IgG within 2 weeks of symptoms, with some as soon as 1 week after initially feeling ill.[18] Further, antibodies from patients with severe illness had the strongest correlation between antibody levels and neutralizing viral response. This pattern, with a vigorous early antibody response, demonstrating stronger neutralization capacity among patients with severe COVID-19, has been duplicated by others and clearly demonstrates an association between severity of illness and early humoral immune response to native infection.[19]

Given this pattern, there has been an appropriate focus on IgG and IgM production over the course of COVID-19 infection; however, antibody levels may not tell the whole story. As noted, higher binding antibody levels have been found among patients suffering from severe, rather than mild, COVID-19 disease.[20] Over the course of one to 6 months, anti-RBD IgG and IgM levels decrease, with an associated 5-fold reduction in plasma neutralizing activity. Importantly, memory B-cells, capable of rapidly producing RBD-specific antibodies, remain unchanged 6 months after infection, indicating the potential for the body to rapidly increase antibody levels on repeat antigen exposure.[21] Further, while IgG and IgM are important neutralizing antibodies (help clear virus by binding to viral receptors and inhibiting viral particles' ability to bind host cells, as well as preventing the uncoating of viral genome in the endosome), IgA predominates in serum, saliva, and bronchoalveolar lavage fluid of patients with SARS-CoV-2. Given the described limitations of the innate immune response in the lower respiratory tract, IgA neutralizing antibodies may play an important role in early response to infection.[22] Less is known about differential IgA response by disease severity, a knowledge gap that, once filled, may help us better understand variations in host response to infection.

The cellular immune response to SARS-CoV-2 also correlates with the severity of COVID-19 illness, however, in an opposite direction than that of humoral immunity. Analysis of blood samples from patients infected with SARS-CoV-2 found that those with mild disease had a robust SARS-CoV-2-specific INF-γ-producing T-cell response against S1, M, and N viral proteins within the first 2 weeks of symptom onset while patients with moderate disease developed cellular responses to these epitopes at a slower rate, reaching equivocal numbers only 3-weeks postsymptom onset. Patients with severe disease had still not started developing high numbers of SARS-CoV-2 specific T-cells by the end of the acute infection follow-up.[18] Fortunately, among those who recover, including recovery from severe disease, 97% maintained detectable SARS-CoV-2-specific memory T-cells out to at least 28 weeks, suggesting that even a delayed cellular response may produce longer lasting immunity across the spectrum of disease severity.[18]

Interestingly, significant peripheral T-cell lymphopenia has been identified as a marker of severe COVID-19 infection. A recent systematic review of the T-cell response to SARS-CoV-2 infection found significantly lower CD3+, CD4+, and CD8+ cell counts in critically ill patients and those who ended up dying of COVID-19 as compared with survivors and moderately ill patients.[23] Further, in a multivariable-adjusted analysis, CD8+ T-cell counts of less than 165 cells/μL were independently associated with COVID-19 related mortality.[24] Similarly, lower helper T-cell levels and higher CD4:CD8 ratios have also been identified as strong predictors of mortality.[25] Dysregulation of the T-regulatory cell (Treg)/Th17 balance has further been implicated in severity of infection, with increased Th17 and decreased Treg cells in patients with severe COVID-19.[26] Treg's play a critical role in dampening an overreactive immune response for the maintenance of immune homeostasis and self-tolerance during viral infections. Th17 cells produce IL-17 which can promote the production of downstream proinflammatory molecules, including IL-1, TNF, IL6, and neutrophil chemoattractants. In the murine model of ARDS, IL-17 has previously been shown to augment lung parenchyma destruction by amplifying proinflammatory mediators and neutrophil recruitment.[27]

In effect, COVID-19 severity of illness demonstrates a dichotomous immune response, with early humoral activation and delayed cellular immune response associated with more severe disease, while early T-cell activation predominates in milder cases (**Fig. 1**).[28] Fortunately, SARS-CoV-2 specific memory B- and T-cells are present following recovery in patients across the spectrum of disease, indicating the potential for a more rapid immune response on future antigenic exposures.

VACCINATION AGAINST SARS-CoV-2

SARS-CoV-2 vaccination is a safe and effective tool for preventing severe illness and death from

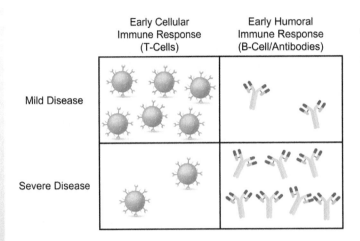

	Early Cellular Immune Response (T-Cells)	Early Humoral Immune Response (B-Cell/Antibodies)
Mild Disease		
Severe Disease		

Fig. 1. Graphical representation of differential humoral and cellular immune response to SARS-CoV-2 infection by disease severity.

COVID-19.[29,30] There are 4 types of vaccines currently approved by the World Health Organization Emergency Use Listing process for the treatment of COVID-19: nucleic acid (BNT162b2/ Pfizer, mRNA 1273/Moderna), nonreplicating viral vector (ChAdOx1 nCoV019/AstraZeneca/Covishield, Ad26.COV2.S/Janssen), inactivated whole virus (BBIBP-CorV/Sinopharm, CoronaVac/ Sinovac, BBV152/Covaxin), and protein subunit (NVX-CoV2373/Novavax).[31] Pfizer, Moderna, and Janssen remain to be the only vaccines with either emergency use or full authorization by the FDA in the United States.[32]

Pfizer and Moderna vaccines carry mRNA, encapsulated in a lipid nanoparticle that encodes a modified version of the SARS-CoV-2 S-protein.[33] This modified mRNA has intentional mutations so translated, the S-protein is in its prefusion conformation, critical for the preservation of neutralization-sensitive epitopes and therefore effective vaccine-induced immunity. In contrast, Janssen's vaccine delivers DNA that codes for the SARS-CoV-2 S-protein on a recombinant adenovirus vector. The DNA is transcribed, producing S-protein, stimulating strong humoral and cellular immune responses.[34,35] Study of the mRNA vaccine platforms to demonstrate successful production of neutralizing antibodies, active SARS-CoV-2 specific CD4+ and CD8+ T-cells, and robust levels of cytokines such as IFNγ.[36] A study of the Pfizer vaccine demonstrated a strong SARS-CoV-2 spike-specific memory B-cell response, peaking 1 week after the second dose, which gradually declined over time but maintained strong ACE2/ RBD binding inhibiting activity for at least 6 months.[37] Such circulating vaccine-induced spike-specific memory B-cells were restimulated *in vitro* and demonstrated ability to differentiate into anti-spike IgG or IgM-secreting cells.

The Pfizer, Moderna, and Janssen vaccines have each shown to be safe and effective at reducing severe COVID-19 illness by 88%, 93%, and 71%, respectively, following 2 doses of the mRNA or one dose of the adenovirus vector vaccine.[29] The Washington State Department of Health has been compiling and releasing data on COVID-19 cases, hospitalizations, and deaths by vaccination status since February 2021. They report that, among 12 to 34 year olds, unvaccinated individuals were 5-times more likely to be hospitalized with COVID-19 compared with their fully vaccinated age-matched counterparts. For those over the age of 65, the risk of COVID-19 hospitalization is 7-fold higher among the unvaccinated, with a risk of death 13-times greater than fully vaccinated individuals in the same age group.[38] Comparably, significant adverse events associated with vaccine were exceedingly rare (between 0.2% and 0.3%).[39] Patients do report symptoms following vaccination, most frequently injection site pain and fatigue or malaise; however, these are overwhelmingly mild and short lasting, with greater than 80% resolving within 2 days.[40]

Dual antigen exposure from both vaccine and infection may also augment the host immune response. Early work comparing serial IgG levels between previously infected and COVID-19 naïve individuals found that IgG levels were similar after 1 mRNA vaccine dose in those with a history of COVID-19 to those following 2 doses in participants without prior infection.[41] Expanding on this work, researchers found that while COVID-19 naïve individuals developed lower overall IgG levels, the 2 groups had comparable neutralizing antibodies and S-specific B-cell levels 8 months after vaccination. Interestingly, the COVID-19 naïve subjects also exhibited higher SARS-CoV-2-specific cytokine production, CD4+ T-cell activation, and proliferation than those who recovered from COVID-19.[42] While the exact mechanism behind the elevated T-cell response following vaccination in COVID-19 individuals remains uncertain, this finding is reassuring, particularly in the setting of the previously noted association of a robust cellular response to infection and the development of only mild symptoms.

As the pandemic has stretched over multiple years, appropriate concern has been directed to the potential of waning immunity following initial vaccination. Marot and colleagues found that neutralizing antibodies against SARS-CoV-2 declined 38.5% among health care workers as soon as 2 months after primary COVID-19 infection and 3 months after the second mRNA vaccine dose.[43] Such declines varied by age and sex, with those over age 65 experiencing a larger decrease in antibody levels following vaccination compared with those between the ages of 18 to 44. Further, vaccine-mediated antibodies among men in this older cohort were found to decrease 46% more than in similarly aged women.[44] Such declines in antibody levels have led the Centers for Disease Control and Prevention, to recommend vaccine boosters and continued use of masks in high-risk areas to limit viral transmission.

There has also been concern that mutations in the S-protein, such as those appreciated in the Omicron variant, may allow the virus to evade neutralization by vaccine-elicited antibodies. To assess this possibility, researchers evaluated the neutralizing capacity of sera collected from individuals recently (<3 months) and remotely (6–12 months) vaccinated with any of the 3 major vaccines available in the United States against wild-type, Delta, and Omicron SARS-CoV-2 variants.[45] They further tested the sera of subjects recently boosted with either mRNA vaccine. While the neutralization of the Omicron variant was not appreciated among those who received only the initial vaccine regimen, neutralization was appreciated using sera from those who received a booster dose. Taken together, and particularly in the setting of recurrent COVID-19 surges, boosters remain a recommended mechanism to increase protection from severe COVID-19 illness.[45]

CLINICAL OUTCOMES OF AN IMBALANCED IMMUNE RESPONSE

While the immune response to COVID-19 facilitates the viral clearance and imparts at least some protection against future infections, an excessively robust response has been implicated as a potential driver of severe disease. Specifically, high levels of cytokines including increases in circulating T-cell chemoattractants, natural killer (NK) cells, macrophages, and classic neutrophils, with an absence of IFN types I and III are found in individuals suffering from severe COVID-19.[46] Such response, paired with elevated IL-6 and IL1RA cytokines suggest a link between COVID-19 and cytokine release syndrome, characterized by vigorous activation of vast numbers of white blood cells resulting in exuberant release of proinflammatory cytokines that in turn activate more white blood cells in a cascading fashion.[23,46,47] High concentrations of IL-6, a proinflammatory cytokine, have also been correlated with lymphopenia, increased severity of disease and mortality.[23,48] Together, local and systemic inflammation, particularly when paired with risk for secondary bacterial infections, increase the risk of progression of disease to ARDS.[49] A review of 72 publications reported that 30% of patients admitted to the ICU with COVID-19 went on to develop lung edema, dyspnea, hypoxemia, or ARDS and 65% of those who developed ARDS died.[49,50] Infection is one of the main inducers of lung edema in ARDS, traditionally known to be caused by neutrophil activation in other illnesses such as influenza. However, given the high rate of ARDS noted, it is uncertain whether SARS-CoV-2 has a unique pathophysiologic immune response that may further predispose to lung injury.[49]

Among the more feared complications of COVID-19 infection are the development of myocarditis and pericarditis. Importantly, while cardiac involvement from COVID-19 infection does occur, clinically significant myocarditis remains a rare complication, with cases typically mild and self-limited.[51,52] In a study of 100 COVID-19 recovered individuals 78% demonstrated myocardial inflammation on cardiac MRI, directly associated with severity of illness, the presence of cardiac symptoms, and time from infection to imaging.[53] Fortunately, most cases are asymptomatic, with an analysis of nearly 1600 COVID-19 positive college athletes finding only 5 who developed cardiac symptoms, although cardiac MRI identified more than 7-times greater number of individuals with evidence of cardiac involvement. Fortunately, all individuals with abnormal cardiac MRIs saw some degree of improvement on serial imaging, again indicating a largely self-limited disease course.[54] In comparison, vaccine-associated myocarditis remains rare. Data from Israel found only 54 cases out of 2.5 million vaccinated individuals, with data from the European Medicines Agency identifying even lower rates of 1.6 per million Pfizer vaccines and 3.0 per million doses of Moderna.[55,56] Cases were predominantly among young or adolescent males, with 76% described as mild. In fact, only 14 individuals in the Israeli data were found to have reduced left ventricular systolic function, with most having recovery of function at follow-up. As opposed to myocarditis, pericarditis has been observed more commonly among older patients and at a later time point with a median of 20 days after the most recent vaccine dose.[51]

Multiple potential immunologic mechanisms have been proposed as drivers of infection and vaccine-associated myocarditis. Specifically following infection, the two-leading hypothesis for the mechanism of myocarditis include direct viral infection of cardiac myocytes and a maladaptive immune response, as described above. Interestingly, histologic analysis of biopsy tissue from patients with SARS-CoV-2 infected myocarditis did not display the classic lymphocytic pattern associated with viral myocarditis. This has led many to believe that overactivation of the immune response, particularly in the setting of severe COVID-19, likely contributes to cardiac dysfunction through thromboinflammation and endothelial dysfunction.[57] Work has also specifically implicated CD68+ T-cells found in high numbers in the myocardium of COVID-19 hearts, in the development of myocarditis following infection.[58] Vaccine-associated myocarditis is thought to result from parallel, though importantly different mechanisms. The previously noted nucleoside modifications to the mRNA vaccines are designed in part to reduce the innate immune system's response to foreign RNA molecules. At least some vaccine-associated myocarditis cases may represent a breakthrough of this innate immune response, a mechanism associated with certain genetic predispositions.[59] Another proposed mechanism evokes molecular mimicry of the S-protein transcribed from the delivered mRNA resulting in cross-reactivity with alpha-myosin.[60] Eosinophilic hypersensitivity has further been implicated as a mechanism particularly given the predilection for second or third dose and been described with the smallpox vaccine, as well.[61] Finally, sex hormones may play a role in the noted male predominance of COVID-19 and vaccine-associated myocarditis. Specifically, estrogen may work to mitigate proinflammatory T-cells, while testosterone may block the function of certain anti-inflammatory cells, allowing for excess immune activation and subsequent myocardial damage.[57]

SUMMARY

The immune response to the novel SARS-CoV-2 virus is pivotal in both regaining health and potentially attenuating the development of severe disease. Early robust humoral response coupled with a delayed cellular immune response is associated with severe disease. Further, dysregulated immune response, including cytokine release syndrome, can lead to worse outcomes, particularly via the development of ARDS. Finally, while rare, infection and vaccine-associated myocarditis can occur, though typically in mild and self-limited forms. Importantly, our understanding of the immune mechanisms underlying health and disease in COVID-19 have been essential to the rapid development of safe and effective vaccines, which remain among our best tools for combating this pandemic.

CLINICS CARE POINTS

- Humoral and cellular immune responses are induced by both natural and vaccine mediated COVID-19 antigenic exposure.
- The balance of early cellular and humoral immune response is associated with the severity of COVID-19 illness.
- Clinically significant COVID-19 vaccine mediated myocarditis is rare.

DISCLOSURE

All others report no conflicts of interest. J.E. Ebinger is supported by grant funding from the NIH/NHLBI (K23-HL153888). B. Weber is supported by grant funding from NHLBI K23 HL15927601, AHA 21CDA851511, and IANC/ASNC 2021 Award.

REFERENCES

1. Organization WH. WHO coronavirus (COVID-19) Dashboard. Available at: https://covid19.who.int. Accessed January 19, 2022.
2. Huang Y, Yang C, Xu X-f, et al. Structural and functional properties of SARS-CoV-2 spike protein: potential antivirus drug development for COVID-19. Acta Pharmacol Sin 2020;41(9):1141–9.
3. Gorbalenya AE, Baker SC, Baric RS, et al. The species Severe acute respiratory syndrome-related coronavirus: classifying 2019-nCoV and naming it SARS-CoV-2. Nat Microbiol 2020;5(4):536–44.
4. Boechat JL, Chora I, Morais A, et al. The immune response to SARS-CoV-2 and COVID-19 immunopathology - Current perspectives. Pulmonology 2021; 27(5):423–37.
5. Hasan MN, Haider N, Stigler FL, et al. The global case-fatality rate of COVID-19 has been declining

since may 2020. Am J Trop Med Hyg 2021;104(6): 2176–84.

6. Wang Q, Zhang Y, Wu L, et al. Structural and functional basis of SARS-CoV-2 entry by using human ACE2. Cell 2020;181(4):894–904.e899.

7. Shang J, Ye G, Shi K, et al. Structural basis of receptor recognition by SARS-CoV-2. Nature 2020; 581(7807):221–4.

8. Thoms M, Buschauer R, Ameismeier M, et al. Structural basis for translational shutdown and immune evasion by the Nsp1 protein of SARS-CoV-2. Science 2020;369(6508):1249–55.

9. Mallinas SR, Maner JK, Ashby Plant E. What factors underlie attitudes regarding protective mask use during the COVID-19 pandemic? Pers Individ Dif 2021;181:111038.

10. Paul E, Steptoe A, Fancourt D. Attitudes towards vaccines and intention to vaccinate against COVID-19: Implications for public health communications. Lancet Reg Health - Europe 2021;1:100012.

11. Zhou L, Ayeh SK, Chidambaram V, et al. Modes of transmission of SARS-CoV-2 and evidence for preventive behavioral interventions. BMC Infect Dis 2021;21(1):496.

12. Sungnak W, Huang N, Bécavin C, et al. SARS-CoV-2 entry factors are highly expressed in nasal epithelial cells together with innate immune genes. Nat Med 2020;26(5):681–7.

13. Alfi O, Yakirevitch A, Wald O, et al. Human nasal and lung tissues infected ex vivo with SARS-CoV-2 Provide Insights into differential tissue-specific and virus-specific innate immune responses in the upper and lower respiratory tract. J Virol 2021;95(14):e0013021.

14. MacMicking JD. Interferon-inducible effector mechanisms in cell-autonomous immunity. Nat Rev Immunol 2012;12(5):367–82.

15. Narayanan K, Huang C, Lokugamage K, et al. Severe acute respiratory syndrome coronavirus nsp1 suppresses host gene expression, including that of type I interferon, in infected cells. J Virol 2008;82(9):4471–9.

16. Vanderheiden A, Ralfs P, Chirkova T, et al. Type I and type III interferons Restrict SARS-CoV-2 infection of human airway epithelial cultures. J Virol 2020;94(19).

17. Carsetti R, Zaffina S, Piano Mortari E, et al. Different innate and adaptive immune responses to SARS-CoV-2 infection of asymptomatic, mild, and severe cases. Front Immunol 2020;11.

18. Almendro-Vázquez P, Laguna-Goya R, Ruiz-Ruigomez M, et al. Longitudinal dynamics of SARS-CoV-2-specific cellular and humoral immunity after natural infection or BNT162b2 vaccination. Plos Pathog 2021;17(12):e1010211.

19. Padoan A, Sciacovelli L, Basso D, et al. IgA-Ab response to spike glycoprotein of SARS-CoV-2 in patients with COVID-19: a longitudinal study. Clin Chim Acta 2020;507:164–6.

20. Liu X, Wang J, Xu X, et al. Patterns of IgG and IgM antibody response in COVID-19 patients. Emerg Microbes Infect 2020;9(1):1269–74.

21. Gaebler C, Wang Z, Lorenzi JCC, et al. Evolution of antibody immunity to SARS-CoV-2. Nature 2021; 591(7851):639–44.

22. Sterlin D, Mathian A, Miyara M, et al. IgA dominates the early neutralizing antibody response to SARS-CoV-2. Sci Transl Med 2021;13(577).

23. Shrotri M, van Schalkwyk MCI, Post N, et al. T cell response to SARS-CoV-2 infection in humans: a systematic review. PLoS One 2021;16(1):e0245532.

24. Luo M, Liu J, Jiang W, et al. IL-6 and CD8+ T cell counts combined are an early predictor of in-hospital mortality of patients with COVID-19. JCI Insight 2020;5(13).

25. Liu Q, Fang X, Tokuno S, et al. Prediction of the clinical outcome of COVID-19 patients using T lymphocyte subsets with 340 cases from Wuhan, China: a retrospective cohort study and a web visualization tool. medRxiv 2020.

26. Xu Z, Shi L, Wang Y, et al. Pathological findings of COVID-19 associated with acute respiratory distress syndrome. Lancet Respir Med 2020;8(4):420–2.

27. Muir R, Osbourn M, Dubois AV, et al. Innate lymphoid cells are the predominant Source of IL-17A during the early Pathogenesis of acute respiratory distress syndrome. Am J Respir Crit Care Med 2016;193(4):407–16.

28. Gao L, Zhou J, Yang S, et al. The dichotomous and incomplete adaptive immunity in COVID-19 patients with different disease severity. Signal Transduction Targeted Ther 2021;6(1):113.

29. Self WH, Tenforde MW, Rhoads JP, et al. Comparative Effectiveness of Moderna, Pfizer-BioNTech, and Janssen (Johnson & Johnson) Vaccines in Preventing COVID-19 Hospitalizations Among Adults Without Immunocompromising Conditions — United States, March—August 2021. MMWR Morb Mortal Wkly Rep 2021;70:1337–1343.

30. Baden LR, El Sahly HM, Essink B, et al. Efficacy and safety of the mRNA-1273 SARS-CoV-2 vaccine. N Engl J Med 2021;384(5):403–16.

31. Organization WH. COVID-19 vaccine Tracker. Available at: https://covid19.trackvaccines.org/agency/who/. Accessed January 30, 2022.

32. Administration UFaD. COVID-19 vaccines. Available at: https://www.fda.gov/emergency-preparedness-and-response/coronavirus-disease-2019-covid-19/covid-19-vaccines. Accessed January 30, 2022.

33. Bettini E, Locci M. SARS-CoV-2 mRNA vaccines: Immunological mechanism and beyond. Vaccines (Basel) 2021;9(2).

34. Custers J, Kim D, Leyssen M, et al. Vaccines based on replication incompetent Ad26 viral vectors: Standardized template with key considerations for a risk/

benefit assessment. Vaccine 2021;39(22): 3081–101.

35. Barouch DH, Stephenson KE, Sadoff J, et al. Durable humoral and cellular immune responses 8 Months after Ad26.COV2.S vaccination. New Engl J Med 2021;385(10):951–3.

36. Sahin U, Muik A, Derhovanessian E, et al. COVID-19 vaccine BNT162b1 elicits human antibody and TH1 T cell responses. Nature 2020;586(7830):594–9.

37. Ciabattini A, Pastore G, Fiorino F, et al. Evidence of SARS-CoV-2-specific memory B cells six Months after vaccination with the BNT162b2 mRNA vaccine. Front Immunol 2021;12.

38. Washington State Department of Health Public Health Outbreak Coordination I, and Surveillance; Disease Control and Health Statistics. COVID-19 cases, hospitalizations, and deaths by vaccination status. January 26, 2022.

39. Beatty AL, Peyser ND, Butcher XE, et al. Analysis of COVID-19 vaccine type and adverse effects following vaccination. JAMA Netw Open 2021; 4(12):e2140364.

40. Ebinger JE, Lan R, Sun N, et al. Symptomology following mRNA vaccination against SARS-CoV-2. Prev Med 2021;153:106860.

41. Ebinger JE, Fert-Bober J, Printsev I, et al. Antibody responses to the BNT162b2 mRNA vaccine in individuals previously infected with SARS-CoV-2. Nat Med 2021;27(6):981–4.

42. Lozano-Rodríguez R, Valentín-Quiroga J, Avendaño-Ortiz J, et al. Cellular and humoral functional responses after BNT162b2 mRNA vaccination differ longitudinally between naive and subjects recovered from COVID-19. Cell Rep 2022;38(2):110235.

43. Marot S, Malet I, Leducq V, et al. Rapid decline of neutralizing antibodies against SARS-CoV-2 among infected healthcare workers. Nat Commun 2021; 12(1):844.

44. Levin EG, Lustig Y, Cohen C, et al. Waning immune humoral response to BNT162b2 Covid-19 vaccine over 6 Months. N Engl J Med 2021;385(24):e84.

45. Garcia-Beltran WF, St Denis KJ, Hoelzemer A, et al. mRNA-based COVID-19 vaccine boosters induce neutralizing immunity against SARS-CoV-2 Omicron variant. Cell 2022;185(3):457–466.e4.

46. Blanco-Melo D, Nilsson-Payant BE, Liu WC, et al. Imbalanced host response to SARS-CoV-2 Drives development of COVID-19. Cell 2020;181(5): 1036–45.e1039.

47. Woodruff MC, Ramonell RP, Nguyen DC, et al. Extra-follicular B cell responses correlate with neutralizing antibodies and morbidity in COVID-19. Nat Immunol 2020;21(12):1506–16.

48. Hadjadj J, Yatim N, Barnabei L, et al. Impaired type I interferon activity and inflammatory responses in severe COVID-19 patients. Science 2020;369(6504): 718–24.

49. Li L, Huang Q, Wang DC, et al. Acute lung injury in patients with COVID-19 infection. Clin Transl Med 2020;10(1):20–7.

50. Boehmer TK, Kompaniyets L, Lavery AM, et al. Association between COVID-19 and myocarditis using hospital-based Administrative data - United States, March 2020-January 2021. MMWR Morb Mortal Wkly Rep 2021;70(35):1228–32.

51. Diaz GA, Parsons GT, Gering SK, et al. Myocarditis and pericarditis after vaccination for COVID-19. JAMA 2021;326(12):1210–2.

52. Mevorach D, Anis E, Cedar N, et al. Myocarditis after BNT162b2 Vaccination in Israeli Adolescents. New England Journal of Medicine 2020;386(10):998–999.

53. Puntmann VO, Carerj ML, Wieters I, et al. Outcomes of Cardiovascular Magnetic Resonance imaging in patients recently recovered from coronavirus disease 2019 (COVID-19). JAMA Cardiol 2020;5(11): 1265–73.

54. Daniels CJ, Rajpal S, Greenshields JT, et al. Prevalence of clinical and Subclinical myocarditis in Competitive athletes with recent SARS-CoV-2 infection: Results from the Big ten COVID-19 cardiac Registry. JAMA Cardiol 2021;6(9):1078–87.

55. Witberg G, Barda N, Hoss S, et al. Myocarditis after Covid-19 vaccination in a Large health Care Organization. New Engl J Med 2021;385(23):2132–9.

56. Lazaros G, Klein AL, Hatziantoniou S, et al. The novel platform of mRNA COVID-19 vaccines and myocarditis: Clues into the potential underlying mechanism. Vaccine 2021;39(35):4925–7.

57. Bozkurt B, Kamat I, Hotez PJ. Myocarditis with COVID-19 mRNA vaccines. Circulation 2021; 144(6):471–84.

58. Fox SE, Falgout L, Vander Heide RS. COVID-19 myocarditis: quantitative analysis of the inflammatory infiltrate and a proposed mechanism. Cardiovasc Pathol 2021;54:107361.

59. Caso F, Costa L, Ruscitti P, et al. Could Sars-coronavirus-2 trigger autoimmune and/or autoinflammatory mechanisms in genetically predisposed subjects? Autoimmun Rev 2020;19(5):102524.

60. Vojdani A, Kharrazian D. Potential antigenic cross-reactivity between SARS-CoV-2 and human tissue with a possible link to an increase in autoimmune diseases. Clin Immunol 2020;217:108480.

61. Murphy JG, Wright RS, Bruce GK, et al. Eosinophilic-lymphocytic myocarditis after smallpox vaccination. Lancet 2003;362(9393):1378–80.

The Direct and Indirect Effects of COVID-19 on Acute Coronary Syndromes

Thomas A. Kite, BM, BS, MRCP[a],*, Susil Pallikadavath[a],
Chris P. Gale, MB BS, PhD, FRCP[b,c,d], Nick Curzen, PhD, FRCP[e],
Andrew Ladwiniec, MA, MD, FRCP[a]

KEYWORDS

- COVID-19 • Acute coronary syndrome • ST-elevation myocardial infarction
- Non–ST-elevation myocardial infarction

KEY POINTS

- The COVID-19 pandemic has resulted in wide-ranging direct and indirect consequences for patients with ACS.
- A sudden, unexpected decline in hospitalizations for ACS and an increase in out-of-hospital deaths coincided with the onset of the COVID-19 pandemic.
- ACS in patients with COVID-19 is associated with excess rates of adverse events, particularly when medical intervention is delayed.
- During the COVID-19 pandemic, many patients with ACS have been required to undergo alternative diagnostic and therapeutic strategies due to reorganization of health care resources.
- Studies to further elucidate the complex relationship between SARS-CoV-2 infection and myocardial injury or infarction are required.

INTRODUCTION

Severe acute respiratory syndrome coronavirus 2 (SARS-CoV-2) has resulted in the most significant infectious disease outbreak and public health emergency for a century. Declared a pandemic by the World Health Organization in March 2020, coronavirus disease 2019 (COVID-19) has infected millions and caused excess mortality and morbidity across the world. Health care systems have been required to restructure and adapt to an entirely novel disease entity, while providing routine and emergency care for existing illness.

Patients with acute coronary syndrome (ACS) provide one such example in which these challenges intersected (**Fig. 1**). The diagnosis and treatment of acute myocardial infarction (MI) has attracted much scientific attention during the COVID-19 pandemic by virtue of several critical issues:

1. An internationally observed reduction in hospital admission rates for ACS[1,2]
2. SARS-CoV-2 infection is associated with myocardial injury,[3] accentuated predominantly in patients with underlying cardiometabolic risk factors[4]

This article originally appeared in Cardiology Clinics, Volume 40, Issue 3, August 2022.
[a] Department of Cardiovascular Sciences and the NIHR Leicester Biomedical Research Centre, Glenfield Hospital, University of Leicester and University Hospitals of Leicester NHS Trust, Groby Road, Leicester, LE3 9QP, United Kingdom; [b] Leeds Institute of Cardiovascular and Metabolic Medicine, University of Leeds, Leeds, LS2 9JT, United Kingdom; [c] Leeds Institute for Data Analytics, University of Leeds, Leeds, LS2 9JT, United Kingdom; [d] Department of Cardiology, Leeds Teaching Hospitals NHS Trust, Great George Street, Leeds, LS1 3EX, United Kingdom; [e] Faculty of Medicine, University of Southampton and University Hospital Southampton NHS Foundation Trust, Tremona Road, Southampton, SO16 6YD, United Kingdom
* Corresponding author.
E-mail address: tom.kite@nhs.net

Heart Failure Clin 19 (2023) 185–196
https://doi.org/10.1016/j.hfc.2022.08.002
1551-7136/23/© 2022 Elsevier Inc. All rights reserved.

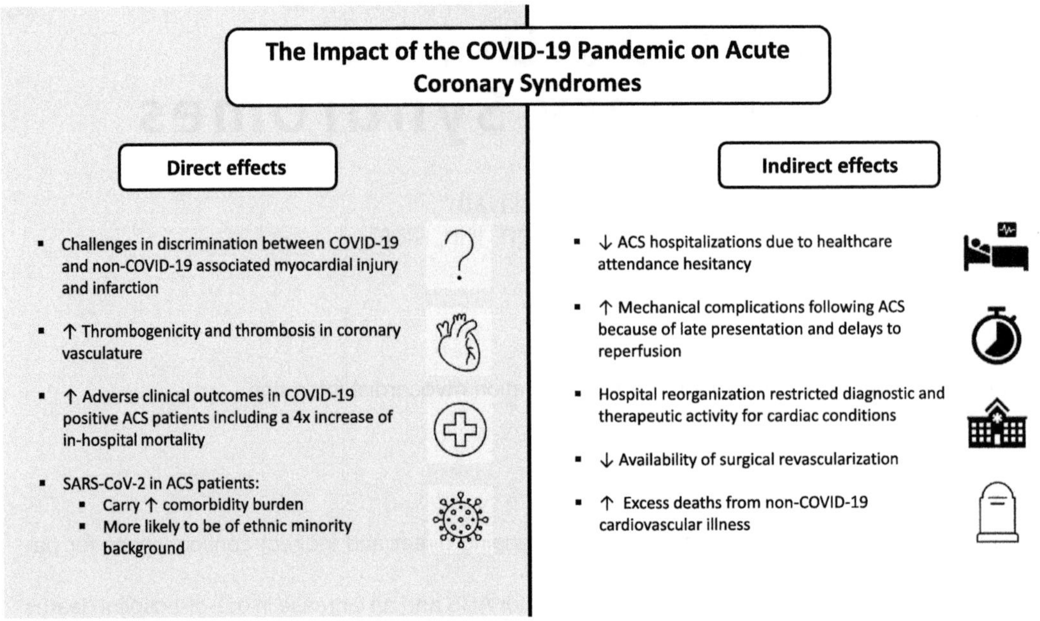

The Impact of the COVID-19 Pandemic on Acute Coronary Syndromes

Direct effects

- Challenges in discrimination between COVID-19 and non-COVID-19 associated myocardial injury and infarction
- ↑ Thrombogenicity and thrombosis in coronary vasculature
- ↑ Adverse clinical outcomes in COVID-19 positive ACS patients including a 4x increase of in-hospital mortality
- SARS-CoV-2 in ACS patients:
  - Carry ↑ comorbidity burden
  - More likely to be of ethnic minority background

Indirect effects

- ↓ ACS hospitalizations due to healthcare attendance hesitancy
- ↑ Mechanical complications following ACS because of late presentation and delays to reperfusion
- Hospital reorganization restricted diagnostic and therapeutic activity for cardiac conditions
- ↓ Availability of surgical revascularization
- ↑ Excess deaths from non-COVID-19 cardiovascular illness

Fig. 1. The direct and indirect effects of the COVID-19 pandemic on patient with acute coronary syndromes.

3. There are perceived diagnostic challenges with discrimination between COVID-19–related and non–COVID-19–related myocardial injury and infarction[5]
4. Health care system reorganization limited the availability of ACS diagnostic tools and therapeutic strategies[6]

The present article addresses these challenges and discusses findings of the International COVID-ACS and UK-ReVasc registries, studies unique in their scope and investigation of the direct and indirect effects of the COVID-19 pandemic on patients with ACS.

COVID-19 AND THE CARDIOVASCULAR SYSTEM: A CHANGING LANDSCAPE

It rapidly became apparent that the SARS-CoV-2 virus would have wide-reaching consequences for patients with cardiovascular disease, because such risk factor profiles were recognized to portend an increased risk of hospitalization and mortality after infection.[7] Yet perhaps more unexpected was the sudden and unheralded decline in cases of heart attack observed at the outset of the COVID-19 pandemic. For example, in one of the first such reports, De Filippo and colleagues documented a 25% reduction in hospital admissions for all ACS in Northern Italy.[2] These data that have since been replicated in larger and more robust analyses that also show preponderance for greater decreases in non–ST-elevation

acute coronary syndrome (NSTE-ACS) presentations.[1,8] Moreover, increases in out-of-hospital cardiac arrest and death at home when compared with prepandemic periods were described, suggesting that many patients were forgoing medical attention.[9,10]

Where did all the heart attacks go? Viral respiratory infections are well recognized to increase the risk of acute MI,[11] so why was this not reflected in greater hospital attendances during the initial waves of the pandemic? Proposed theories comprised: (1) a desire from patients to self-manage symptoms at home (perhaps compounded by societal pressures to quarantine), (2) a reduction in activity levels that may provoke MI, or (3) a fear of COVID-19 contagion in health care settings.[12]

Against the backdrop of falling heart attack case rates, a story of the complex interplay between SARS-CoV-2 infection and cardiovascular disease developed, fueled by rapid dissemination of knowledge via social media platforms.[13] Case series described spontaneous and excess microthrombi and macrothrombi development in multiple vascular beds,[14] myocarditis masquerading as ST-elevation myocardial infarction (STEMI),[15] and elevated rates of myocardial injury in patients with COVID-19 infection.[16]

However, the exact degree and frequency of acute myocardial injury in patients with COVID-19, and its relationship with the cardiovascular system, has been difficult to accurately define. In perhaps the most robust study to investigate its prevalence, Lala and colleagues reported acute myocardial injury by means of cardiac troponin elevation in 36% of 2736 patients hospitalized with COVID-19.[17] Elevated levels correlated with disease severity, as troponin concentrations 3 times the upper reference limit were associated with a 3-fold increased risk of mortality.[17] Multiple hypotheses have been presented for the direct impact of SARS-CoV-2 on the cardiovascular system, ranging from supply-demand mismatch-mediated ischemia, intravascular thrombosis and endotheliitis, systemic hypoxia, or direct viral insult and injury—each a result of a systemic inflammatory cascade as the SARS-CoV-2 viral spike protein binds to angiotensin-converting enzyme 2 receptors.[18,19] Indeed, discrimination between COVID-19–related and non–COVID-19–related myocardial injury has been intensely debated and acknowledged to present significant diagnostic and therapeutic uncertainty for frontline clinicians.[20]

An important group comprises those patients who present with ACS while concurrently infected with COVID-19. Such cases were documented in early observations to experience greater rates of adverse outcomes.[21] The worse clinical courses may be explained by:

1. Direct pathophysiological consequences of SARS-CoV-2 infection that may lead to an increased propensity for plaque rupture and thrombus propagation[22] and/or,
2. Indirect patient and system-related factors that created delay in receipt of timely medical care.

It became clear that descriptive and mechanistic observational studies were required to better understand this multifaceted disease process.

ACUTE CORONARY SYNDROME AND CONCOMITANT COVID-19: THE INTERNATIONAL COVID-ACS REGISTRY

The International COVID-ACS Registry was designed to evaluate the characteristics and outcomes of ACS patients with concurrent COVID-19 infection.[23] As it became clear that this population represented a unique challenge,[24] the study was established in March 2020 to elucidate potential mechanisms that may account for the adverse outcomes observed.

The International COVID-ACS Registry has provided a pragmatic means of investigator-initiated data collection via an online web-hosted portal. Lead investigators were cognisant of increased clinical demands, redeployed research personnel, and redistributed funding streams during this period. The criteria for study inclusion were as follows: (1) COVID-19 positive (or high index suspicion according to clinical status and chest imaging findings[25]) and (2) invasive coronary angiography undertaken for suspected ACS.

A consortium of international investigators collected data from 144 STEMI and 121 NSTE-ACS patients with concomitant COVID-19 infection. The key findings of the study were consistent regardless of ACS subtype (**Table 1**).[23] Compared with pre-COVID-19 control cohorts taken from the UK-based British Cardiovascular Intervention Society (BCIS) National PCI Audit,[26] and English data from the Myocardial Ischaemia National Audit Project (MINAP) databases,[27] COVID-19 positive ACS patients had:

1. A greater burden of comorbidity
2. Longer delays seeking medical attention, and, in the case of STEMI, less frequently received timely reperfusion therapy
3. Higher rates of intensive care unit admission for ventilatory and/or hemodynamic support
4. Greater adverse in-hospital clinical events, including a more than doubling of cardiogenic shock
5. A 4-fold increase of in-hospital mortality

These results have been replicated in similar observational studies that have described in-hospital mortality rates of 23% to 33% in COVID-19 positive STEMI patients, and the predilection for SARS-CoV-2 infection in ACS patients with greater baseline comorbidities and of minority ethnic background (**Table 2**).[28,29] Furthermore, elevated rates of unfavorable presenting characteristics such as out-of-hospital cardiac arrest, heart failure, and cardiogenic shock in COVID-19–positive STEMI patients have consistently been described in the literature.[23,28–30]

The principal mechanistic finding of the International COVID-ACS Registry was that time taken for patients to render the hospital was prolonged when compared with pre-COVID controls, and that this was associated with poorer clinical outcomes (symptom onset to admission: COVID-STEMI vs controls: median 339.0 minutes vs 173.0 minutes; $P < .001$; COVID NSTE-ACS vs controls: 417.0 minutes vs 295.0 minutes; $P = .012$). In addition, a lengthening of door-to-balloon time in the STEMI subgroup was also observed (COVID-STEMI vs controls: median 83.0 minutes vs 37.0 minutes; $P < .001$). These delays to reperfusion have also been noted in analyses of COVID-19–negative patients hospitalized with STEMI,[31,32] thereby suggesting that pathways and well-established systems of care struggled to adapt to the obligatory organizational

Table 1
Summary of key findings from the International COVID-ACS registry

	COVID-STEMI (n = 144)	Pre-COVID-19 STEMI Controls (n = 24,961)	COVID NSTE-ACS (n = 121)	Pre-COVID NSTE-ACS Controls (n = 46,389)
Baseline Characteristics				
Mean age, y (SD)	64 (13)	66 (13)	67 (13)	70 (13)
Male	78%	72%	79%	66%
Hypertension	65%	45%	68%	58%
Hyperlipidemia	46%	29%	63%	34%
Diabetes mellitus	34%	21%	39%	31%
Chronic kidney disease	10%	4%	20%	10%
Symptom onset to admission, min (IQR)	339.0 (175.0–1481.5)	173.0 (107.0–387.0)	417.0 (157.0–2904.0)	295.0 (130.0–1021.0)
Door-to-balloon time, min (IQR)	83.0 (37.0–336.0)	37.0 (31.0–109.0)	-	-
Postprocedure				
ICU admission	46%	NA	34%	NA
Ventilation	21%	4%	12%	0.4%
Pressor support	27%	5%	19%	0.9%
Mechanical support device	6%	3%	0.8%	0.6%
In-hospital outcomes				
Death	23%	6%	7%	1%
Myocardial infarction	6%	NA	4%	NA
Stent thrombosis	1%	NA	0%	NA
Bleeding	3%	0.3%	3%	0.1%
Stroke	2%	0.1%	0.8%	0.1%
Cardiogenic shock	20%	9%	5%	1%
Length of hospital stay, d (IQR)	6.5 (2.7–12.7)	3.0 (2.0–5.0)	6.9 (3.4–18.4)	5.0 (3.0–8.0)

Pre-COVID-19 STEMI controls were taken from the British Cardiovascular Intervention Society 2018 to 2019 National Audit database. Pre-COVID-19 NSTE-ACS controls were taken from the Myocardial Ischaemia National Audit Project 2019 database.

Abbreviations: IQR, interquartile range; NA, data not available; NSTE-ACS, non–ST-elevation acute coronary syndrome; SD, standard deviation; STEMI, ST-elevation myocardial infarction.

Adapted from Kite TA, Ludman PF, Gale CP, et al. International Prospective Registry of Acute Coronary Syndromes in Patients With COVID-19. *J Am Coll Cardiol.* 2021;77(20):2466-2476.

changes, screening of patients, and preparation of personnel in the catheter laboratory. Such insights in STEMI patients, irrespective of COVID-19 status, provide valuable information and add credence to early hypotheses that deferment in seeking and receiving medical care may, in part, explain the excess mortality rates observed. Public health communications that requested the public "stay at home," alongside a perceived fear of COVID-19 contagion, appear to have impacted patterns of health care–seeking behavior.

Studies to date have often focused on COVID-19–positive patients with STEMI. The unique scope of the International COVID-ACS registry also afforded insights into patients with NSTE-ACS who underwent an invasive strategy. A striking observation existed that magnitude increases of cardiogenic shock and in-hospital mortality compared with prepandemic controls were similar across both COVID-19–positive ACS subgroups (see **Table 1**). It is well-established that superior outcomes after STEMI are driven by a time-critical concept dependent on expeditious mechanical reperfusion of an occluded coronary artery. For NSTE-ACS, however, the underlying pathophysiology differs and the association with

Table 2
Key characteristics and outcomes of COVID-19–positive ACS registry studies

Study	Duration	Design	Size	Inclusion Criteria	Comparator Group	Treatment Delays	Diabetes Mellitus	OHCA	Cardiogenic Shock	In-Hospital Mortality	Other Key Findings
International COVID-ACS Registry Kite et al,[23] 2021	March 2020 – July 2020	Prospective, multicenter, international	144 STEMI, 121 NSTE-ACS	Only if underwent invasive angiography	Pre-COVID-19 BCIS and MINAP databases	Yes	36%	STEMI: 9% NSTE-ACS: 1%	STEMI: 20% NSTE-ACS: 5%	STEMI:23% NSTE-ACS: 7%	• High comorbidity burden in both ACS subgroups • Prolonged length of hospital stay in COVID-19–positive patients
NACMI Registry Garcia et al,[28] 2021	January 2020 – December 2020	Prospective, multicenter, United States & Canada	230 STEMI	Invasive angiography and medically managed patients	Historical propensity-matched cohort from Midwest STEMI Consortium	Yes	46%	11%	18%	33%	• COVID-19–positive patients more likely to be of minority ethnic origin • Lower rate of angiography in COVID-19–positive patients

(continued on next page)

Table 2
(continued)

Study	Duration	Design	Size	Inclusion Criteria	Comparator Group	Treatment Delays	Diabetes Mellitus	OHCA	Cardiogenic Shock	In-Hospital Mortality	Other Key Findings
Spanish Infarct Code Registry Rodriguez-Leor et al,[30] 2021	March 2020 – April 2020	Retrospective, multicenter, Spain	91 STEMI	Invasive angiography and medically managed patients	Contemporary COVID-19–negative controls	No	23%	8%	10%	23%	• COVID-19–positive patients more likely to undergo mechanical thrombectomy and receive GPIIb/IIIa inhibitors • COVID-19–positive patients had higher rates of in-hospital stent thrombosis

MINAP registry Rashid et al,[29] 2021	March 2020 – May 2020	Retrospective, multicenter, England	153 STEMI, 311 NSTE-ACS	Angiography and medically managed patients	Contemporary COVID-19 negative controls	Yes	38%	Combined STEMI/NSTE-ACS: 4%	Combined STEMI/NSTE-ACS: 10%	Combined STEMI/NSTE-ACS: 24%	• High comorbidity burden in both ACS subgroups • COVID-19–positive patients more likely to be of minority ethnic origin • Lower rate of angiography in COVID-19–positive patients

Abbreviations: ACS, acute coronary syndrome; BCIS, British Cardiovascular Intervention Society; MINAP, Myocardial Ischaemia National Audit Project; NACMI, North American COVID-19 Myocardial Infarction; NSTE-ACS, non–ST-elevation acute coronary syndrome; OHCA, out-of-hospital cardiac arrest; STEMI, ST-elevation myocardial infarction.

time from symptom onset to angiography (with or without revascularization) is not nearly as strong when compared with STEMI.[33] Although limited by a small number of events in the NSTE-ACS group, acceptance that a median time difference of approximately 2 hours until attendance at hospital between COVID-19–positive NSTE-ACS and pre–COVID-19 control patients would result in such marked differences in outcome is initially problematic. Although confounding factors could be at play, in a cohort of patients who carry a greater comorbidity burden (especially those with concomitant COVID-19 in the COVID-ACS registry),[34] the direct effect of COVID-19 infection could be playing a greater part in this ACS subgroup. Worse outcomes in COVID-19–positive NSTE-ACS patients have been associated with excess thrombogenicity, comparable to reports in COVID-19 positive STEMI cases.[22] This concept surely warrants further investigation.[35]

PERCUTANEOUS CORONARY INTERVENTION IN PATIENTS TYPICALLY TREATED WITH CORONARY ARTERY BYPASS GRAFTING: THE UK-ReVasc REGISTRY

Beyond the direct effects of SARS-CoV-2 infection on the global population, the COVID-19 pandemic continues to indirectly impact on mortality and morbidity. Specifically, health care system reorganization, together with changes in patient and clinician behavior, have resulted in restricted access to previously established care pathways, with suggestions that this has led to an increase in deaths from cardiovascular disease.[36]

In particular, reduced availability of intensive care unit support for procedures such as coronary artery bypass grafting (CABG) and valvular surgery resulted in an up to 80% reduction in cardiac surgical activity during the first wave of the COVID-19 pandemic.[37] In the United Kingdom, National Health Service resources were largely reconfigured to only provide care for emergency cases, with clinicians requested to defer treatment for all other patients in preparation for the expected surge of patients with COVID-19 who would require hospitalization and ventilatory support.[38]

The UK-ReVasc Registry was therefore established as a prospective multicenter registry to investigate the characteristics and outcomes of patients with patterns of coronary artery disease (CAD) that in ordinary circumstances would have been deemed most suitable for CABG surgery,[39] but who were instead treated with percutaneous coronary intervention (PCI) because of pandemic-enforced constraints on surgical activity and access to ventilators.[40]

The registry reported on 215 patients (75% of whom presented with NSTE-ACS) from across the UK and found in-hospital major adverse cardiovascular events were no different when compared with a conventional pre–COVID-19 all-comer PCI population from the British Cardiovascular Intervention Society (BCIS) National Audit database, despite greater complexity of CAD and a more comorbid population in the UK-ReVasc Registry. Low rates of death, MI, stroke, and unplanned revascularization in the registry population persisted out to 30 days follow-up. When compared with isolated CABG data from the United Kingdom, in-hospital mortality was similar, although lower rates of major bleeding and shorter length of hospital stay were observed in the UK-ReVasc Registry group.

To the best of our knowledge, the UK-ReVasc Registry is the only prospective study that has collected data on this specific and novel patient cohort who were required to undergo an alternative mode of revascularization due to the impact of the COVID-19 pandemic. It affords examination of contemporary PCI techniques in a group of patients with high rates of multivessel disease (96%) and left main stem disease (52%), that according to international guidelines should primarily be reserved for CABG.[41]

Even so, only short-term outcomes have been reported and initial findings perhaps generate more questions than answers. In a population with anatomically complex CAD, does revascularization with contemporary PCI techniques provide comparable and durable longer-term results that are comparable to CABG surgery? Have calcium modification techniques and newer generation drug-eluting stents evolved such that historical revascularization trials require updating to best inform current practice? Longer-term follow-up is required, and ongoing, to inform these important discussions.

DISCUSSION

As we enter the next stages of the COVID-19 pandemic, with decreasing rates of mortality driven by improved therapeutics and mass vaccination strategies, now seems an appropriate juncture to reflect on the impact of this unprecedented crisis. Focus must now shift away from COVID-19 itself and examine the consequences of the SARS-CoV-2 virus on other areas of health service delivery and care.

Cardiovascular disease remains the leading cause of morbidity and mortality globally and is associated with 17.8 million deaths annually.[42] Patients with cardiovascular disease have been one of the hardest hit groups during the pandemic period, directly because of SARS-CoV-2 predilection to cause severe infection and death in people with such comorbidities, but also indirectly because of restricted availability and access to routine and urgent health care provision that is recognized to improve clinical outcomes.[6] These 2 effects are well illustrated by the International COVID-ACS and UK-ReVasc registries.[23,39]

Governments and public health institutions mandated their citizens to stay at home and reduce social interaction to avoid contagion, particularly those of older age and at high risk of complications after SARS CoV-2 infection.[43] Yet, it is this group of individuals, in whom the cardiovascular disease is most prevalent,[44] that will have been disadvantaged the most from delays in receiving timely diagnosis and treatment.[45] For instance, surges in mechanical complications after ACS have been described during the pandemic, with reports of ventricular septal and free wall rupture,[46,47] acute functional mitral regurgitation,[48] and cardiogenic shock not seen in such frequency since before the establishment of primary PCI networks.[49]

Perhaps the most noteworthy impact of the pandemic has yet to be quantified. Concerns regarding the provision of care for noncommunicable diseases such as cardiovascular disease and cancer have been raised, but arguably overlooked because of the imminent threat of COVID-19–positive patients overwhelming acute hospitals. Although some patients were able to undergo an alternative treatment strategy, many have been left struggling to access timely and appropriate health care. Analyses from electronic health record and mortality in England estimate that up to 100,000 excess deaths from indirect effects of the COVID-19 pandemic have occurred in patients with cardiovascular disease, predominantly due to reduced supply of, and demand for, cardiac services.[50] Beyond this, we are only beginning to see the repercussions of delayed and suboptimal revascularization in patients with ACS that will lead to larger infarct size, adverse ventricular remodeling, heart failure, and arrhythmias.[51]

Despite the immeasurable suffering caused by COVID-19, it remains remarkable that in the face of adversity health care systems and professionals have remained resilient despite these unprecedented challenges. The 2 multicenter registries presented in this report are examples of the clinical and research communities collaborating to better understand the implications of COVID-19 for patients with ACS. Despite the stark messages delivered, they highlight areas that require further focus and investigation to ensure improved care for our patients. Future concerted research initiatives, support from national political leaders, and robust public education campaigns are therefore required to ameliorate the adverse direct and indirect impact caused by the ongoing COVID-19 pandemic.

SUMMARY

The COVID-19 pandemic has proven a "double threat" to patients with ACS. First, the complex interplay of direct SARS-CoV-2 infection, diagnostic uncertainty in the acute setting, and time delays to hospital in this population have contributed to excess morbidity and mortality. Second, a shift of attention and resource from established service pathways to focus on the surges of COVID-19–positive patients requiring emergency care has required modification of traditionally accepted treatment approaches. Given recent acknowledgment that SARS-CoV-2 endemicity is now inevitable,[52] improved public health messaging and adaptation of existing health care systems to provide optimal treatment to both COVID-19 and non–COVID-19 patients is required. Future clinical research initiatives to better understand the COVID-19 and multiple mechanistic factors at play in patients with ACS are essential.

TRIBUTE TO PROFESSOR TONY GERSHLICK

Finally, this article would be incomplete without remembrance of Professor Tony Gershlick, pioneer interventional cardiologist, esteemed clinical trialist, revered mentor, and friend to many who died of COVID-19 in November 2020. The chief investigator of both the COVID-ACS and UK-ReVasc registry studies, Tony's passion for research over a long and distinguished career has resulted in a remarkable impact on cardiovascular care in the United Kingdom and beyond.

CLINICS CARE POINTS

This article focuses on the indirect and direct effects of the COVID-19 pandemic on the diagnosis, treatment, and outcomes of patients with ACS. The following points should be considered by care providers when approaching this important patient population:

- In COVID-19–positive patients, discrimination between ACS and acute myocardial injury is a challenge. In hospitalized COVID-19 patients, elevated cardiac enzymes occur in approximately one-third and portend an increased risk of morbidity and mortality.

- Patients with ACS are more likely to experience delays in receipt of timely care during the COVID-19 pandemic because of changes in health care–seeking behavior and care pathway modifications.

- As compared with pre–COVID-19 cohorts, STEMI and NSTE-ACS patients with concomitant COVID-19 infection experience greater rates of in-hospital bleeding, stroke, cardiogenic shock, and mortality. Delayed medical intervention appears to be a significant mechanistic factor.

- Owing to the indirect effect of the COVID-19 pandemic on health care delivery, many patients with ACS have undergone alternative revascularization strategies (eg, PCI rather than CABG). Short-term outcomes are robust but follow-up of such cohorts is necessary to establish whether long-term clinical outcomes are acceptable.

- The direct and indirect effects of the COVID-19 pandemic on patients with ACS have yet to be precisely defined. Future investigations should aim to understand the complex interplay of SARS-CoV-2 infection and MI. Understanding and addressing the indirect impact of COVID-19 on patients with established cardiovascular disease is of critical importance to optimize care and improve outcomes.

DISCLOSURE

C.P. Gale reports personal fees from AstraZeneca, Amgen, Bayer, Boehringer-Ingelheim, Daiichi Sankyo, Vifor Pharma, Menarini, Wondr Medical, Raisio Group, and Oxford University Press; grants from BMS, Abbott, British Heart Foundation, National Institute for Health Research, Horizon 2020, and ESC, outside the submitted work. N. Curzen reports unrestricted research grants from Boston Scientific, HeartFlow, and Beckman Coulter, and speaker/consultancy fees from Boston, Abbott, and HeartFlow outside the submitted work. The remaining authors have no conflicts of interest to declare.

REFERENCES

1. Mafham MM, Spata E, Goldacre R, et al. COVID-19 pandemic and admission rates for and management of acute coronary syndromes in England. Lancet 2020;396(10248):381–9.
2. De Filippo O, D'Ascenzo F, Angelini F, et al. Reduced rate of hospital admissions for ACS during Covid-19 outbreak in Northern Italy. N Engl J Med 2020;383(1):88–9.
3. Bonow RO, Fonarow GC, O'Gara PT, et al. Association of coronavirus disease 2019 (COVID-19) with myocardial injury and mortality. JAMA Cardiol 2020;5(7):751–3.
4. Richardson S, Hirsch JS, Narasimhan M, et al. Presenting characteristics, Comorbidities, and outcomes Among 5700 patients hospitalized with COVID-19 in the New York city area. JAMA 2020;323(20):2052–9.
5. Sandoval Y, Januzzi JL Jr, Jaffe AS. Cardiac troponin for Assessment of myocardial injury in COVID-19: JACC review Topic of the Week. J Am Coll Cardiol 2020;76(10):1244–58.
6. Ball S, Banerjee A, Berry C, et al. Monitoring indirect impact of COVID-19 pandemic on services for cardiovascular diseases in the UK. Heart 2020;106(24):1890–7.
7. Zhou F, Yu T, Du R, et al. Clinical course and risk factors for mortality of adult inpatients with COVID-19 in Wuhan, China: a retrospective cohort study. Lancet 2020;395(10229):1054–62.
8. Garcia S, Albaghdadi MS, Meraj PM, et al. Reduction in ST-segment elevation cardiac Catheterization Laboratory Activations in the United States during COVID-19 pandemic. J Am Coll Cardiol 2022;77(16):1994–2003.
9. Rashid M, Gale CP, Curzen N, et al. Impact of COVID19 pandemic on the incidence and management of out of hospital cardiac arrest in patients presenting with acute myocardial infarction in England. J Am Heart Assoc 2020;9(22):e018379.
10. Wu J, Mamas MA, Mohamed MO, et al. Place and causes of acute cardiovascular mortality during the COVID-19 pandemic. Heart 2020;107(2):113–9.
11. Kwong JC, Schwartz KL, Campitelli MA. Acute myocardial infarction after Laboratory-Confirmed Influenza infection. N Engl J Med 2018;378(26):2540–1.
12. Krumholz H. Where have all the heart attacks gone? New York Times 2020.
13. Aggarwal NR, Alasnag M, Mamas MA. Social media in the era of COVID-19. Open Heart 2020;7(2).
14. Klok FA, Kruip M, van der Meer NJM, et al. Incidence of thrombotic complications in critically ill ICU patients with COVID-19. Thromb Res 2020;191:145–7.
15. Doyen D, Moceri P, Ducreux D, et al. Myocarditis in a patient with COVID-19: a cause of raised troponin and ECG changes. Lancet 2020;395(10235):1516.
16. Shi S, Qin M, Shen B, et al. Association of cardiac injury with mortality in hospitalized patients with COVID-19 in Wuhan, China. JAMA Cardiol 2020;5(7):802–10.
17. Lala A, Johnson KW, Januzzi JL, et al. Prevalence and impact of myocardial injury in patients hospitalized with COVID-19 infection. J Am Coll Cardiol 2020;76(5):533–46.

18. Akhmerov A, Marban E. COVID-19 and the heart. Circ Res 2020;126(10):1443–55.
19. Libby P, Luscher T. COVID-19 is, in the end, an endothelial disease. Eur Heart J 2020;41(32): 3038–44.
20. Giustino G, Pinney SP, Lala A, et al. Coronavirus and cardiovascular disease, myocardial injury, and arrhythmia: JACC focus Seminar. J Am Coll Cardiol 2020;76(17):2011–23.
21. Stefanini GG, Montorfano M, Trabattoni D, et al. ST-elevation myocardial infarction in patients with COVID-19: clinical and angiographic outcomes. Circulation 2020;141(25):2113–6.
22. Choudry FA, Hamshere SM, Rathod KS, et al. High thrombus burden in patients with COVID-19 presenting with ST-elevation myocardial infarction. J Am Coll Cardiol 2020;76(10):1168–76.
23. Kite TA, Ludman PF, Gale CP, et al. International prospective registry of acute coronary syndromes in patients with COVID-19. J Am Coll Cardiol 2021; 77(20):2466–76.
24. Bangalore S, Sharma A, Slotwiner A, et al. ST-Segment elevation in patients with Covid-19 - a case series. N Engl J Med 2020;382(25):2478–80.
25. Simpson S, Kay FU, Abbara S, et al. Radiological society of North America Expert Consensus Statement on reporting chest CT findings related to COVID-19. Endorsed by the society of Thoracic Radiology, the American College of Radiology, and RSNA - secondary Publication. J Thorac Imaging 2020;35(4):219–27.
26. Ludman P. British Cardiovascular Intervention Society database: insights into interventional cardiology in the United Kingdom. Heart 2019;105(16):1289.
27. Wilkinson C, Weston C, Timmis A, et al. The myocardial Ischaemia national Audit Project (MINAP). Eur Heart J Qual Care Clin Outcomes 2020;6(1):19–22.
28. Garcia S, Dehghani P, Grines C, et al. Initial findings from the North American COVID-19 myocardial infarction registry. J Am Coll Cardiol 2021;77(16): 1994–2003.
29. Rashid M, Wu J, Timmis A, et al. Outcomes of COVID-19-positive acute coronary syndrome patients: a multisource electronic healthcare records study from England. J Intern Med 2021;290(1):88–100.
30. Rodriguez-Leor O, Cid Alvarez AB, Perez de Prado A, et al. In-hospital outcomes of COVID-19 ST-elevation myocardial infarction patients. EuroIntervention 2021;16(17):1426–33.
31. De Luca G, Verdoia M, Cercek M, et al. Impact of COVID-19 pandemic on mechanical reperfusion for patients with STEMI. J Am Coll Cardiol 2020; 76(20):2321–30.
32. Xiang D, Xiang X, Zhang W, et al. Management and outcomes of patients with STEMI during the COVID-19 pandemic in China. J Am Coll Cardiol 2020; 76(11):1318–24.
33. Ting HH, Chen AY, Roe MT, et al. Delay from symptom onset to hospital presentation for patients with non-ST-segment elevation myocardial infarction. Arch Intern Med 2010;170(20):1834–41.
34. McManus DD, Gore J, Yarzebski J, et al. Recent trends in the incidence, treatment, and outcomes of patients with STEMI and NSTEMI. Am J Med 2011;124(1):40–7.
35. Matsushita K, Hess S, Marchandot B, et al. Clinical features of patients with acute coronary syndrome during the COVID-19 pandemic. J Thromb Thrombolysis 2021;52(1):95–104.
36. Wadhera RK, Shen C, Gondi S, et al. Cardiovascular deaths during the COVID-19 pandemic in the United States. J Am Coll Cardiol 2021;77(2):159–69.
37. Mohamed Abdel Shafi A, Hewage S, Harky A. The impact of COVID-19 on the provision of cardiac surgical services. J Card Surg 2020;35(6):1295–7.
38. NHS England. Next steps on NHS response to COVID-19: Letter from Sir Simon Stevens and Amanda Pritchard. 2020. Available at: https://www.england.nhs.uk/coronavirus/wp-content/uploads/sites/52/2020/03/20200317-NHS-COVID-letter-FINAL.pdf. Accessed 10th September 2021.
39. Kite TA, Ladwiniec A, Owens CG, et al. Outcomes following PCI in CABG candidates during the COVID-19 pandemic: the prospective multicentre UK-ReVasc registry. Catheter Cardiovasc Interv 2021;99(2):305–13.
40. Harky A, Harrington D, Nawaytou O, et al. COVID-19 and cardiac surgery: the perspective from United Kingdom. J Card Surg 2020;36(5):1649–58.
41. Neumann FJ, Sousa-Uva M, Ahlsson A, et al. 2018 ESC/EACTS Guidelines on myocardial revascularization. Eur Heart J 2019;40(2):87–165.
42. Group WCRCW. World Health Organization cardiovascular disease risk charts: revised models to estimate risk in 21 global regions. Lancet Glob Health 2019;7(10):e1332–45.
43. World Health Organization. Coronavirus disease (COVID-19) advice for the public. 2020. Available at: https://www.who.int/emergencies/diseases/novel-coronavirus-2019/advice-for-public. Accessed 13 October 2021.
44. Bae S, Kim SR, Kim MN, et al. Impact of cardiovascular disease and risk factors on fatal outcomes in patients with COVID-19 according to age: a systematic review and meta-analysis. Heart 2021;107(5):373–80.
45. Kiss P, Carcel C, Hockham C, et al. The impact of the COVID-19 pandemic on the care and management of patients with acute cardiovascular disease: a systematic review. Eur Heart J Qual Care Clin Outcomes 2021;7(1):18–27.
46. Alsidawi S, Campbell A, Tamene A, et al. Ventricular septal rupture complicating delayed acute myocardial infarction presentation during the COVID-19 pandemic. JACC Case Rep 2020;2(10):1595–8.

47. Albiero R, Seresini G. Subacute left ventricular free wall rupture after delayed STEMI presentation during the COVID-19 pandemic. JACC Case Rep 2020;2(10):1603–9.

48. Kunkel KJ, Anwaruddin S. Papillary Muscle rupture due to delayed STEMI presentation in a patient self-Isolating for Presumed COVID-19. JACC Case Rep 2020;2(10):1633–6.

49. Moroni F, Gramegna M, Ajello S, et al. Collateral Damage: medical care avoidance behavior Among patients with myocardial infarction during the COVID-19 pandemic. JACC Case Rep 2020;2(10):1620–4.

50. Banerjee A, Chen S, Pasea L, et al. Excess deaths in people with cardiovascular diseases during the COVID-19 pandemic. Eur J Prev Cardiol 2021;28(14):1599–609.

51. Sutton MG, Sharpe N. Left ventricular remodeling after myocardial infarction: pathophysiology and therapy. Circulation 2000;101(25):2981–8.

52. Phillips N. The coronavirus is here to stay - here's what that means. Nature 2021;590(7846):382–4.

A Review of ST-Elevation Myocardial Infarction in Patients with COVID-19

Nima Ghasemzadeh, MD[a], Nathan Kim, MD[b], Shy Amlani, MD[c],
Mina Madan, MD, MHS[d], Jay S. Shavadia, MD[e], Aun-Yeong Chong, MD[f],
Alireza Bagherli, MD[g], Akshay Bagai, MD, MHS[h], Jacqueline Saw, MD[i],
Jyotpal Singh, MSc[j], Payam Dehghani, MD[j,*]

KEYWORDS

- ST-Elevation myocardial infarction • COVID-19 • SARS-COV 2

KEY POINTS

- COVID-19 leads to a hyper-inflammatory response and increase in procoagulants and platelet activation predisposing to an acute myocardial infarction (AMI).
- Cardiogenic shock is more common in patients with COVID-19 who present with STEMI than those without COVID-19 but not cardiac arrest
- STEMI in patients with COVID-19 is associated with worse clinical outcomes compared with STEMI in patients without COVID-19.
- Primary PCI remains the first-line treatment approach in patients with COVID-19 who develop STEMI

INTRODUCTION

The Coronavirus disease 2019 (COVID-19) pandemic has led to a significant increase in worldwide morbidity and mortality. Patients with COVID-19 are at risk for developing a variety of cardiovascular conditions including acute coronary syndromes, stress-induced cardiomyopathy, and myocarditis. Patients with COVID-19 who develop ST-elevation myocardial infarction (STEMI) are at a higher risk of morbidity and mortality when compared with their age- and sex-matched STEMI patients without COVID-19.[1] We review current knowledge on the pathophysiology of STEMI in patients with COVID-19, clinical presentation, outcomes, and the effect of the COVID-19 pandemic on overall STEMI care.

EPIDEMIOLOGY

Initial reports suggested a drop in the number of patients presenting with STEMI to hospitals in the few months following February–March 2020.[2–11] However, some centers later witnessed a U-shaped phenomenon in STEMI incidence during the pandemic.[12,13] This U-shaped phenomenon

This article originally appeared in Cardiology Clinics, Volume 40, Issue 3, August 2022.

[a] Georgia Heart Institute, Gainesville, GA 30501, USA; [b] Northeast Georgia Health System, Gainesville, GA 30501, USA; [c] William Osler Health System, Brampton, 2100 Bovaird Drive East, Ontario L6R 3J7, Canada; [d] Schulich Heart Centre, Sunnybrook Health Sciences Centre, 2075 Bayview Avenue, Toronto, Ontario M4N 3M5, Canada; [e] Royal University Hospital, Saskatchewan Health, University of Saskatchewan Saskatoon, 103 Hospital Drive, Saskatchewan S7N 0W8, Canada; [f] University of Ottawa Heart Institute, 40 Ruskin Street, Ottawa, Ontario K1Y 4W7, Canada; [g] Windsor Regional Hospital, 1030 Ouellette Avenue, Windsor, Ontario N9A 1E1, Canada; [h] Terrence Donnelly Heart Centre, St. Michael's Hospital, University of Toronto, 30 Bond Street, Toronto, Ontario M5B 1W8, Canada; [i] Vancouver General Hospital, Vancouver, 12th Avenue, Vancouver, British Columbia V5Z 1M9, Canada; [j] Prairie Vascular Research Inc, Regina, 1440 14 Avenue, Saskatchewan S4P 0W5, Canada
* Corresponding author. Prairie Vascular Research Inc, Regina, 1440 14 Avenue, Saskatchewan S4P 0W5, Canada.
E-mail address: pdehghani@me.com

Heart Failure Clin 19 (2023) 197–204
https://doi.org/10.1016/j.hfc.2022.08.007
1551-7136/23/© 2022 Elsevier Inc. All rights reserved.

indicated a decline in STEMI incidence during the first few weeks of the pandemic followed by a rebound in the following weeks.

PATHOPHYSIOLOGY

COVID-19 is caused by SARS-CoV-2 and has been shown to predispose patients to a prothrombotic state, involving both the venous and arterial circulations as well as both microvascular and macrovascular systems.[14,15] This prothrombotic state has been shown to be associated with poor prognosis in patients with COVID-19 pneumonia.[16] Several mechanisms are believed to play a role in this process including inflammation, endothelial dysfunction, and platelet activation (**Fig. 1**).[17] SARS-CoV-

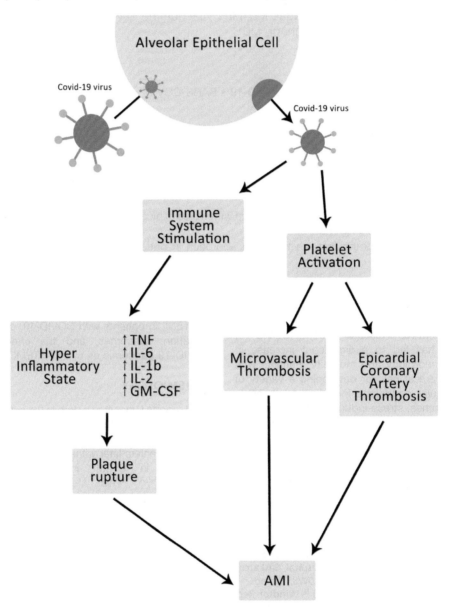

Fig. 1. Pathophysiology of STEMI in patients with COVID-19. COVID-19 induced hyperinflammatory state and thrombosis as mechanisms leading to acute myocardial infarction. COVID-19 enters alveolar epithelial cells via the angiotensin-converting enzyme-2 receptor. Once it gets replicated in these cells, then it exits the alveolar cells and stimulates a dysregulated immune response which leads to hyperinflammatory response with the elevation of multiple biomarkers such as TNF, Interleukin-1 beta (IL-1β), Interleukin-6 (IL-6), interleukin-2 (IL-2), and granulocyte monocyte colony-stimulating factor (GM-CSF). Parallel to this, there is upregulation of procoagulants and increased platelet activation which leads to thrombosis. Hyperinflammatory response and thrombosis are the main mechanisms behind STEMI in patients with COVID-19.

2 infects epithelial respiratory cells by binding to the angiotensin-converting enzyme-2 receptor, viral shedding follows, which stimulates an inflammatory response leading in some cases to a cytokine storm mediated by proinflammatory cytokines such as interleukin 1-β (iL-1 β), iL-2, iL-6, tumor necrosis factor (TNF), and granulocyte macrophage colony-stimulating factor (GM-CSF). This cascade then leads to an overexpression of procoagulant factors such as tissue factor, factor VIII, p-selectin, Von Willebrand factor (vWF), fibrinogen, and down-regulation of anticoagulants which leads to thrombus formation.[18]

A pathologic analysis of 40 hearts from hospitalized patients in Italy who succumbed to COVID-19 showed that 35% of these patients had evidence of myocardial necrosis. The most common reason for myocardial necrosis was the presence of microthrombi, which were distinctly different in composition from thrombus aspirates from epicardial coronary arteries containing more fibrin and terminal complement.[19,20]

PATIENT CHARACTERISTICS

Most of the patients with COVID-19 who presented with STEMI were male in both the Israeli and North American cohorts (**Table 1**).[1,20] Their age ranged from 56 to 75 years.[1] Patients with COVID-19 who presented with STEMI had a significantly lower risk factor burden compared with those who were admitted with STEMI before the COVID-19 pandemic.[20] Most of those patients belonged to racial minorities (23% Hispanics, 24% Blacks, 6% Asians). The most common presenting symptom was dyspnea and 46% of patients had the presence of pulmonary infiltrate on chest x ray.[1] An Italian cohort in Lombardy showed that 85.7% of patients with STEMI experienced myocardial infarction as the first manifestation of COVID-19 and a quarter of those patients reported dyspnea as the initial complaint.[21] Cardiogenic shock is more frequent in patients with COVID-19.[1,9,22]

PROCEDURAL CHARACTERISTICS

In the North American experience, about a quarter of patients with COVID-19 or suspected of having COVID-19 who presented with STEMI did not undergo emergent coronary angiography.[1] Door to balloon (D2B) time was reported in several studies to be significantly longer in patients with COVID-19 compared with historical controls. In a recent meta-analysis of 19 studies mainly across Asia, Europe, and Canada, the mean D2B time was reported to be 8.1 minutes longer in patients with COVID-19 compared with controls.[23] This difference was more noticeable in the North American

Table 1
Comparison of baseline characteristics reported in prior studies

	Garcia et al,[1] 2021	De Luca et al,[9] 2021	Hamadeh et al.[36]	Fardman et al,[13] 2020	Controls Midwest STEMI Consortium
Median Age (y)	65	64	65	62	62
Male Sex (%)	71	73.7	63	81	71
Hypertension (%)	73	54.7	73	52	69
Dyslipidemia (%)	46	41.5	92	58	60
Diabetes mellitus (%)	46	21.8	27	31	28
Prior PCI (%)	13	12.6	—	—	26
Prior MI (%)	13	9.4	—	18	24
Prior CABG (%)	5	1.7	11	2.6	8
Smoking (%)	44	41	—	49	59
Prior stroke/TIA (%)	10	—	8	5.9	9
History of CAD (%)	24	—	78	—	31
Aspirin (%)	38	—	22	—	39
Statin (%)	39	—	42	—	35
Cardiogenic Shock (%)	18	7.7	–	–	10
Out of hospital cardiac arrest (%)	11	6.6			7

Abbreviations: CABG, coronary artery bypass grafting; MI, myocardial infarction; TIA, transient ischemic attack; PCI, percutaneous coronary intervention.

centers with a mean difference of 12 minutes.[1] Patients with COVID-19 presenting with STEMI were more likely to receive medical therapy alone compared with controls (20% vs 2%) and less likely to undergo primary PCI (71% vs 93%). These patients were more likely to have no identifiable culprit lesion on coronary angiography as compared with the control group (23% vs 1%).[1]

In a meta-analysis of several studies, post-PCI thrombolysis-in-myocardial-infarction (TIMI) flow grade was 60% more likely to be suboptimal with TIMI flow less than 3 than the control group of patients from the prepandemic era.[23] Even though left ventricular ejection fraction (LVEF) following primary PCI was reported to be similar in the North American experience, several other studies have shown a significantly lower LVEF (−4.2%) following primary PCI in patients with COVID-19 compared with their counterparts (**Table 2**).[23]

LENGTH OF HOSPITAL STAY

Patients with STEMI who underwent PCI during the pandemic had an overall longer duration of hospital stay as shown in several studies. In the North American experience, the average length of hospital stay was 4 days longer in patients with COVID-19 compared with patients without COVID-19.[1] Other studies have shown an increased length of ICU stay in patients with STEMI who were admitted during the pandemic era as compared with those admitted before the pandemic onset.[23]

IN-HOSPITAL OUTCOMES

In the North American experience, the primary composite endpoint of in-hospital death, stroke, recurrent MI, or repeat revascularization was significantly higher in patients with COVID-19 compared with patients without COVID-19 (36% vs 5%, $P < .001$).[1] This was primarily due to markedly higher risk of in-hospital death in patients with COVID-19 as compared with controls (33% vs 4%, $P < .001$) The incidence of stroke was also statistically higher in patients with COVID-19 (3% vs 0%, $P = .017$). In a meta-analysis conducted by Chew and colleagues, the overall mortality of patients with STEMI was 27% higher during the pandemic as compared with prepandemic controls.[23] Similarly, the Israeli experience reported an overall higher composite endpoint of malignant arrhythmia, congestive heart failure, or in-hospital mortality in those admitted with STEMI in the pandemic era as compared with prepandemic controls (12% vs 8.6%, $P = .04$), **Table 3**.[20] In a large recent retrospective analysis of both out-of-hospital and in-hospital patients with STEMI with COVID-19, the mortality rate was significantly higher when compared with their COVID-19 negative propensity-matched counterparts (15.2% vs 11.2%). In this study, Saad and colleagues also compared the outcomes between in-hospital patients with STEMI with concomitant COVID-19 to in-hospital patients with STEMI without COVID-19 from prior years and reported a dramatically

Table 2
Comparison of procedural characteristics reported in prior studies

	Garcia et al,[1] 2021	De Luca et al,[9] 2021	Fardman et al,[13] 2020	Controls from Midwestern STEMI Consortium
No angiography (%)	22	–	2	0
D2B time, min. Median (IQR)	79 (52–125)	34 (21–36)	52 (29–90)	66 (46–93)
D2B time <90 (%)	58	—	–	73
LV Ejection Fraction (%)	45	–	45	45
Primary PCI (%)	71	–	87	93
Presence of culprit lesion (%)				
Multiple culprits	16	–	6.4	–
No culprit	23	–	–	0
TIMI flow post-PCI (%)				
0–1	6	–	–	2
2–3	94	92.2	–	98
Length of hospital stay, days	6	–	4	2

Abbreviation: D2B, door to balloon time; LV, left ventricular; PCI, percutaneous coronary intervention; TIMI, thrombolysis-in-myocardial-infarction.

Table 3
Comparison of clinical outcomes reported in prior studies

	Garcia et al,[1] 2021	De Luca et al,[9] 2021	Fardman et al,[13] 2020	Controls from Midwestern STEMI Consortium
In-hospital death (%)	33	29	18	5
Stroke (%)	3	–	1.2	0
Recurrent myocardial infarction (%)	2	–	3	0
Unplanned revascularization (%)	4	–	–	4

higher mortality rate of 76% as compared with 44% in those without COVID-19.[24]

DISPARITIES IN ST-ELEVATION MYOCARDIAL INFARCTION MANAGEMENT IN THE COVID-19 ERA

Several studies have shown higher cardiovascular disease-related deaths in the COVID-19 era in racial and ethnic minorities including African Americans, Asians, and Hispanics compared with Whites.[25,26] In a retrospective study of 73,746 patients admitted with AMI in the pandemic and prepandemic eras in the United Kingdom, there was a significantly higher odds ratio of AMI in ethnic minority groups as compared with Whites.[26] These patients, however, were more likely to be younger, male, with lower body mass index, and a higher prevalence of comorbidities. They were more likely to present with out of hospital cardiac arrest (7.6% vs 6.2%, $P = .04$) and cardiogenic shock (3.5% vs 2.4%, $P < .001$) as compared with Whites. There was a longer delay in reperfusion therapy in the minority group as compared with Whites with an absolute increase of 30 minutes in the D2B time.[26] The ethnic minorities were significantly less likely to be discharged on dual antiplatelet therapy compared with Whites (70% vs 73%, $P = .03$). Risk of in-hospital and 7-day mortality was significantly higher in the ethnic subgroup compared with Whites.[26]

REPERFUSION STRATEGIES

Even though primary PCI has been the first-line reperfusion strategy for patients with STEMI in the United States, the rate of fibrinolysis-focused reperfusion strategy remains about 2%-13% nationally.[27] During the COVID-19 pandemic, longer delays were reported to reperfusion. Tim and colleagues reported longer delays of symptom onset to first medical contact (318 vs 82.5 minutes), D2B time (110 vs 84.5 minutes), and catheterization laboratory to balloon time (33 vs 20.5 minutes)

compared with the prepandemic era.[28] Delayed presentation, lack of adequate COVID-19 testing early on, potential hazard to staff members, longer assessment times in emergency departments resulting in longer D2B times and therefore, potentially loss of primary PCI benefit, led to suggestions for a fibrinolytic-first approach in a selected patients with STEMI.[29] However, given the higher rate of no culprit including microthrombi with slow flow, stress-induced cardiomyopathy, COVID-19 induced myocarditis, or pericarditis, fibrinolysis may not only provide no benefit, but confer additional bleeding risk. With the adoption of enhanced safety measures in cardiac catheterization laboratories, greater access to rapid testing, and wider availability of personal protective equipment for staff, a joint recommendation from the ACC, SCAI, and American College of Emergency Physicians (ACEP) later recommended primary PCI for all patients with definite STEMI regardless of COVID-19 diagnosis.[30] Thrombolysis was instead recommended for patients with STEMI with severe COVID-19 pneumonia or those for whom transfer to PCI-capable hospital is not possible within 120 minutes from first medical contact.[30,31]

IMPACT OF COVID-19 PANDEMIC ON SYSTEMS OF CARE IN ST-ELEVATION MYOCARDIAL INFARCTION MANAGEMENT

The COVID-19 pandemic has impacted the delivery of health care in all its aspects around the globe. STEMI systems of care that require a synchronized network of referring hospitals, emergency departments, and PCI-capable cardiac catheterization laboratories have similarly been affected. During the initial phase of the pandemic, some studies suggested up to 31% reduction in cardiac catheterization laboratory activations with an estimated 18% to 20% reduction in primary PCI volume.[11] During the same period, a study by Garcia and colleagues showed an increase of 20% in D2B times as compared with before the pandemic.[11] Several factors were reported to contribute to the increase in time to reperfusion during the pandemic including overwhelmed emergency rooms, COVID-19 testing requirement in the ED before transfer to catheterization laboratory, use of strict infection control measures, and increased use of imaging to triage these patients.[32] Early in the pandemic, it was observed that the time from onset of symptoms to assessment in ED was significantly longer compared with prepandemic times.[23] Fear of exposure to COVID-19 in hospitals and concern for overburdening hospital systems were contributing factors.[33,34] Furthermore, other key challenges in caring for these patients has been shortage of ICU beds and medical equipment such as ventilators, mechanical circulatory support devices, and lack of sufficient health human resources to care for these patients. With the adoption of protocols endorsed by cardiovascular societies and with wider access to COVID-19 testing, some of these challenges have been overcome. Furthermore, triage of patients with low-risk STEMI to non-ICU settings has been proposed to mitigate the challenge of ICU bed shortages. Risk scores such as CADILLAC and Zwolle have been validated in the non–COVID-19 setting to be useful in triage of patients with low-risk STEMI and theoretically were even more needed during the pandemic.[35]

SUMMARY

The COVID-19 pandemic presented a profound international crisis that has altered the landscape of medicine. From disease pathophysiology to the disruption of health care resources, COVID-19 presents unique challenges in terms of the direct and indirect effects on patient care. The pandemic highlights critical stress points within the health care system forcing organizations to reassess resource allocation and management. Patients with STEMI are uniquely affected as this patient population shares special disease characteristics and requires the coordination of multidisciplinary teams involved in STEMI systems of care. We have highlighted these challenges and lessons learned in STEMI management in the face of this pandemic. Overall patients with STEMI with COVID-19 have been shown in several studies to have worse in-hospital outcomes as compared with their COVID-19 negative counterparts. Previously reported racial and ethnic disparities in cardiovascular outcomes are magnified in the face of the pandemic. Further research needs to be conducted to understand the effect of COVID-19 on long-term outcomes of patients with STEMI who survive hospital discharge.

CLINICS CARE POINTS

- Healthcare professionals should be aware that patients presenting with COVID-19 and STEMI have a different presentation profile and disease course in-hospital. Patients with STEMI and COVID-19 tend to have greater mortality rates, lengthier stays at the ICU, and ethnic minorities appear to be disproportionately affected as compared to those without COVID-19.

- Patients with STEMI are uniquely affected as this patient population shares special disease characteristics. More mechanistic studies including ECG and angiogram characteristics are required to better understand different outcomes in this patient population.

- STEMI care has been greatly impacted by COVID-19, with delayed presentation, lack of adequate COVID-19 testing early on, potential hazard to staff members, and longer assessment times in emergency departments resulting in longer D2B times. However, primary PCI should remain the primary focus in this patient population.

ACKNOWLEDGMENTS

We would like to thank all site contributors and the executive leadership of the NACMI registry. We would also like to thank the Saskatchewan Health Research Foundation for their funding support (#5391) in Saskatchewan, Canada.

DISCLOSURE

The authors have nothing to disclose.

REFERENCES

1. Garcia S, Dehghani P, Grines C, et al. Initial Findings from the North American COVID-19 Myocardial Infarction Registry. J Am Coll Cardiol 2021;77(16): 1994–2003.
2. Zitelny E, Newman N, Zhao D. STEMI during the COVID-19 pandemic - an Evaluation of incidence. Cardiovasc Pathol 2020;48:107232.
3. Schiavone M, Gobbi C, Biondi-Zoccai G, et al. Acute coronary syndromes and Covid-19: Exploring the Uncertainties. J Clin Med 2020;9(6).
4. Lauridsen MD, Butt JH, Ostergaard L, et al. Incidence of acute myocardial infarction-related cardiogenic shock during corona virus disease 19 (COVID-19) pandemic. Int J Cardiol Heart Vasc 2020;31:100659.

5. De Rosa S, Spaccarotella C, Basso C, et al. Reduction of hospitalizations for myocardial infarction in Italy in the COVID-19 era. Eur Heart J 2020;41(22): 2083–8.

6. Metzler B, Siostrzonek P, Binder RK, et al. Decline of acute coronary syndrome admissions in Austria since the outbreak of COVID-19: the pandemic response causes cardiac collateral damage. Eur Heart J 2020;41(19):1852–3.

7. De Filippo O, D'Ascenzo F, Angelini F, et al. Reduced rate of hospital admissions for ACS during Covid-19 outbreak in Northern Italy. N Engl J Med 2020;383(1):88–9.

8. Tan W, Parikh RV, Chester R, et al. Single center trends in acute coronary syndrome volume and outcomes during the COVID-19 pandemic. Cardiol Res 2020;11(4):256–9.

9. De Luca G, Verdoia M, Cercek M, et al. Impact of COVID-19 pandemic on mechanical reperfusion for patients with STEMI. J Am Coll Cardiol 2020; 76(20):2321–30.

10. Garcia S, Albaghdadi MS, Meraj PM, et al. Reduction in ST-Segment elevation cardiac catheterization laboratory activations in the United States during COVID-19 pandemic. J Am Coll Cardiol 2020; 75(22):2871–2.

11. Garcia S, Stanberry L, Schmidt C, et al. Impact of COVID-19 pandemic on STEMI care: an expanded analysis from the United States. Catheter Cardiovasc Interv 2021;98(2):217–22.

12. Fabris E, Bessi R, De Bellis A, et al. COVID-19 impact on ST-elevation myocardial infarction incidence rate in a Italian STEMI network: a U-shaped curve phenomenon. J Cardiovasc Med (Hagerstown) 2021;22(5):344–9.

13. Fardman A, Oren D, Berkovitch A, et al. Post COVID-19 acute myocardial infarction rebound. Can J Cardiol 2020;36(11). 1832 e1815-1832 e1816.

14. Wichmann D, Sperhake JP, Lutgehetmann M, et al. Autopsy Findings and venous Thromboembolism in patients with COVID-19: a Prospective cohort study. Ann Intern Med 2020;173(4):268–77.

15. Levi M, Thachil J, Iba T, et al. Coagulation abnormalities and thrombosis in patients with COVID-19. Lancet Haematol 2020;7(6):e438–40.

16. Tang N, Li D, Wang X, et al. Abnormal coagulation parameters are associated with poor prognosis in patients with novel coronavirus pneumonia. J Thromb Haemost 2020;18(4):844–7.

17. Bikdeli B, Madhavan MV, Jimenez D, et al. COVID-19 and thrombotic or Thromboembolic disease: Implications for Prevention, Antithrombotic therapy, and Follow-up: JACC state-of-the-Art review. J Am Coll Cardiol 2020;75(23):2950–73.

18. Chan NC, Weitz JI. COVID-19 coagulopathy, thrombosis, and bleeding. Blood 2020;136(4): 381–3.

19. Pellegrini D, Kawakami R, Guagliumi G, et al. Microthrombi as a major Cause of cardiac Injury in COVID-19: a pathologic study. Circulation 2021; 143(10):1031–42.

20. Fardman A, Zahger D, Orvin K, et al. Acute myocardial infarction in the Covid-19 era: incidence, clinical characteristics and in-hospital outcomes-A multicenter registry. PLoS One 2021;16(6):e0253524.

21. Stefanini GG, Montorfano M, Trabattoni D, et al. ST-elevation myocardial infarction in patients with COVID-19: clinical and angiographic outcomes. Circulation 2020;141(25):2113–6.

22. Popovic B, Varlot J, Metzdorf PA, et al. Changes in characteristics and management among patients with ST-elevation myocardial infarction due to COVID-19 infection. Catheter Cardiovasc Interv 2021;97(3):E319–26.

23. Chew NWS, Ow ZGW, Teo VXY, et al. The global effect of the COVID-19 pandemic on STEMI care: a systematic review and meta-analysis. Can J Cardiol 2021;37(9):1450–9.

24. Saad M, Kennedy KF, Imran H, et al. Association between COVID-19 diagnosis and in-hospital mortality in patients hospitalized with ST-Segment elevation myocardial infarction. JAMA 2021; 326(19):1940–52.

25. Wadhera RK, Figueroa JF, Rodriguez F, et al. Racial and ethnic disparities in heart and Cerebrovascular disease deaths during the COVID-19 pandemic in the United States. Circulation 2021;143(24): 2346–54.

26. Rashid M, Timmis A, Kinnaird T, et al. Racial differences in management and outcomes of acute myocardial infarction during COVID-19 pandemic. Heart 2021;107(9):734–40.

27. Roe MT, Messenger JC, Weintraub WS, et al. Treatments, trends, and outcomes of acute myocardial infarction and percutaneous coronary intervention. J Am Coll Cardiol 2010;56(4):254–63.

28. Tam CF, Cheung KS, Lam S, et al. Impact of coronavirus disease 2019 (COVID-19) outbreak on outcome of myocardial infarction in Hong Kong, China. Catheter Cardiovasc Interv 2021;97(2): E194–7.

29. Welt FGP, Shah PB, Aronow HD, et al. Catheterization laboratory Considerations during the coronavirus (COVID-19) pandemic: from the ACC's interventional Council and SCAI. J Am Coll Cardiol 2020;75(18):2372–5.

30. Mahmud E, Dauerman HL, Welt FGP, et al. Management of acute myocardial infarction during the COVID-19 pandemic: a Position Statement from the society for cardiovascular angiography and interventions (SCAI), the American College of Cardiology (ACC), and the American College of emergency Physicians (ACEP). J Am Coll Cardiol 2020;76(11): 1375–84.

31. Szerlip M, Anwaruddin S, Aronow HD, et al. Considerations for cardiac catheterization laboratory procedures during the COVID-19 pandemic perspectives from the society for cardiovascular angiography and interventions emerging leader Mentorship (SCAI ELM) members and Graduates. Catheter Cardiovasc Interv 2020;96(3):586–97.

32. Bangalore S, Sharma A, Slotwiner A, et al. ST-segment elevation in patients with Covid-19 - a case Series. N Engl J Med 2020;382(25):2478–80.

33. Roffi M, Guagliumi G, Ibanez B. The Obstacle Course of reperfusion for ST-Segment-elevation myocardial infarction in the COVID-19 pandemic. Circulation 2020;141(24):1951–3.

34. Piccolo R, Bruzzese D, Mauro C, et al. Population trends in rates of percutaneous coronary revascularization for acute coronary syndromes associated with the COVID-19 outbreak. Circulation 2020; 141(24):2035–7.

35. Lopez JJ, Ebinger JE, Allen S, et al. Adapting STEMI care for the COVID-19 pandemic: the case for low-risk STEMI triage and early discharge. Catheter Cardiovasc Interv 2021;97(5):847–9.

36. Hamadeh A, Aldujeli A, Briedis K, et al. Characteristics and Outcomes in Patients Presenting With COVID-19 and ST-Segment Elevation Myocardial Infarction. Am J Cardiol 2020;131:1–6.

Mechanical Circulatory Support in COVID-19

Kari Gorder, MD[a],*, Wesley Young, BS[a], Navin K. Kapur, MD[b], Timothy D. Henry, MD[a,c], Santiago Garcia, MD[d], Raviteja R. Guddeti, MD[d], Timothy D. Smith, MD[a]

KEYWORDS

- COVID-19 • Cardiogenic shock • Mechanical circulatory support
- Extracorporeal membrane oxygenation • Acute respiratory distress syndrome

KEY POINTS

- Patients with cardiogenic shock or acute respiratory distress syndrome experience high rates of morbidity and mortality
- Concomitant COVID-19 infection significantly increases risks of complication and death for these patient populations
- The application of mechanical circulatory support technology for patients with COVID-19 infection has the potential to save lives but also brings with it high rates of complications and mortality
- Careful patient selection, diligent management, and a team-based approach are critical to improving outcomes in this challenging patient population
- More research is needed to improve our understanding of which subset of COVID-19 patients may benefit from cardiopulmonary mechanical support

INTRODUCTION

Cardiogenic shock (CS), a devastating complication of acute myocardial infarction (AMI) and other cardiac disorders, is a state of end-organ dysfunction that occurs in the setting of inadequate cardiac output. Despite advances in diagnostic technology, upfront revascularization strategies, and aggressive medical management, CS remains a highly morbid condition fraught with complications and high rates of mortality.[1–3] Mechanical circulatory support (MCS)—to include percutaneous right- and left-ventricular support devices, including extracorporeal membrane oxygenation (ECMO)—offers an additional level of support for select patients, but a standardized approach to the application of this technology remains

challenging, partially due to the inherent difficulties with randomized controlled trials in this heterogeneous and complex patient population.[4,5] However, observational and cohort data from several institutions have shown the utility of the thoughtful application of MCS technology based on objective criteria, invasive monitoring devices, and a multidisciplinary shock team approach.[6,7] The range and diversity of MCS devices has ushered in a new era for patients with CS, but recently clinicians have been faced with a new challenge: a global pandemic. Coronavirus disease 2019 (COVID-19) has challenged our understanding of cardiopulmonary physiology and brought with it unique challenges in a resource-limited environment. Although the primary effect of COVID-19 is on the respiratory system, its deleterious

This article originally appeared in Cardiology Clinics, Volume 40, Issue 3, August 2022.

[a] The Christ Hospital Heart and Vascular Institute, 2139 Auburn Avenue, Cincinnati OH 45219, USA; [b] Tufts Medical Center, 800 Washington Street, Boston, MA 02111, USA; [c] The Carl and Edyth Lindner Center for Research and Education, The Christ Hospital, Cincinnati, OH 45219, USA; [d] Minneapolis Heart Institute, 800 East, 28th Street, Minneapolis, MN 55407, USA
* Corresponding author.
E-mail address: kari.gorder@thechristhospital.com
Twitter: @karigorder (K.G.); @wesyoungpa (W.Y.); @HenrytTimothy (T.D.H.); @RavitejaGuddeti (R.R.G.); @TimDSmithMD (T.D.S.)

consequences have the potential to reach across all organ systems and can adversely affect cardiac function. This review article focuses on our current understanding of the effects of COVID-19 in the adult population as it pertains to CS, the assessment and evaluation of these patients, and the implementation of MCS in patients with cardiac or pulmonary failure, to include both venoarterial (VA) and venovenous (VV) ECMO.

PATHOPHYSIOLOGY AND EPIDEMIOLOGY

Although the pulmonary complications are well-described,[8] COVID-19's deleterious effects are not limited to the lungs. Any organ system, including the cardiac and vascular systems, can be involved, and the presentation of a patient with COVID-19 is often heterogeneous. Although overall rare, patients with COVID-19 can and do experience cardiovascular complications without concomitant pulmonary disease, and it is been shown that COVID-19 patients with underlying cardiovascular comorbidities experience increased morbidity and mortality.[9] Direct cardiovascular complications may occur in isolation, but it is also not uncommon that shock in the setting of COVID-19 is multifactorial and occurs on a spectrum, and includes noncardiac sources of cardiovascular collapses, such as inflammatory and distributive shock.

COVID-19's direct effects on the cardiovascular system are myriad and can include myocardial ischemia, direct cardiomyocyte injury (eg, myocarditis), or isolated right ventricular dysfunction. Although not fully understood, proposed mechanisms for ischemia in COVID-19 patients include virus-mediated macrocirculatory and microcirculatory thrombosis, endothelial dysfunction, and hypercoagulability,[10,11] and can cause a similar phenotype of CS as is seen with classical AMI.[12] Although rare, COVID-19 infection is associated with an increased risk of myocarditis, and in extreme cases can lead to CS refractory to medical management alone.[13–15] Right ventricular (RV) dysfunction, the most common cardiac manifestation of COVID-19 infection in some studies,[16] may be due to the indirect effects of hypoxia, pulmonary emboli, or primarily elevated pulmonary vascular resistance, and can lead to isolated RV failure or biventricular failure (see David W. Louis and colleagues' article, "The Cardiovascular Manifestations of COVID-19," in this issue).

Although most patients with COVID-19 may not experience these complications—or will remain relatively asymptomatic from cardiac complaints[17]—, for select patients, COVID-19 can lead to or precipitate refractory CS. For patients presenting with acute coronary syndrome, the presence of concomitant COVID-19 infection confers a significantly increased risk: patients are presenting later, have a higher risk of developing shock, and have a significantly higher mortality rate. In one prospective registry study, mortality for patients with concurrent COVID-19 and ST-segment elevation myocardial infarction (STEMI) approached 23%, compared with a non-COVID risk of approximately 5%, conferring an odds ratio of 3.33.[18] In the same registry, CS occurred 20% of the time in COVID-19 STEMI patients, compared with 8.7% in controls. The results of the North American COVID-19 ST-Segment Elevation Myocardial Infarction (NACMI) registry were even more sobering: COVID-19 patients presenting with an STEMI experienced a 33% mortality rate, compared with 4% seen in non-COVID-19 controls, with a significantly increased rate of CS at 18%.[19] Although the cause for this disparity is unclear, proposed mechanisms include delayed presentation secondary to reluctance to go to the hospital during a pandemic, prolonged ischemic time, and potentially intrinsic factors of COVID-19 infection, including proinflammatory and prothrombotic effects. Looking at all patients with COVID-19, despite being the most infrequent etiology of shock seen in admitted patients, CS portends the highest mortality of any shock state.[20] As such, its timely recognition, diagnosis, and treatment remain of utmost importance, especially within a cohort of patients critically ill with COVID-19.

DIAGNOSIS AND INITIAL MANAGEMENT OF COVID-19 PATIENTS WITH REFRACTORY CARDIOGENIC SHOCK

Although there is some variability in definition, the diagnosis of CS is classically described as systolic hypotension (SBP < 90 mm Hg or the use of vasopressors) in conjunction with signs of end-organ hypoperfusion in the setting of a reduced cardiac index of less than 2.2 L/min and an elevated pulmonary capillary wedge pressure of greater than 15 mm Hg.[3,21,22] This definition does not describe all phenotypes of CS, and, if stringently applied, may not capture all COVID-19 patients with CS, who may be more likely to present with lower filling pressures due to concomitant distributive shock.[20] For all patients, alternate surrogate markers of shock may be useful, such as cardiac power output or pulmonary artery pulsatility index, and use of the Society for Cardiovascular Angiography and Intervention (SCAI) classification scheme for CS should be considered.[4,5,22,23] Regardless, the diagnosis of CS often requires both noninvasive and invasive hemodynamic assessment, including the placement of a pulmonary artery catheter, which has been shown to improve outcomes in patients with CS.[7] Given the relative infrequence of CS as an etiology of shock in the undifferentiated patient—especially for those patients critically ill with COVID-19—a high index of suspicion for a cardiac etiology of hemodynamic instability is of the utmost importance on the part of the clinician.

As randomized clinical trial data for the application of MCS in COVID-19 patients are sorely lacking, extrapolation from the traditional body of evidence for the application of MCS in CS is necessary. For COVID-19 patients experiencing AMI, early revascularization and standard medical therapy is warranted. For AMI and other etiologies of CS, subsequent medical management may include treating the precipitating insult as well as the use of volume expansion or the addition of vasopressors or inotropes. However, for many patients with CS of any etiology, medical management alone is not sufficient.[5] The decision to escalate to mechanical support for a patient with CS, as well as the selection of a device platform, may be both institution- and patient-specific. Patients with CS may present with isolated left or right ventricular failure, biventricular failure, or have challenges with oxygenation. Options for MCS include the intra-aortic balloon pump (IABP; Getinge, Sweden; Teleflex, Wayne, PA), percutaneous left ventricular assist devices such as the Impella (Abiomed, Danvers, MA), right ventricular support devices with or without oxygenators, and VA ECMO. Algorithms have been proposed to help standardize and guide the application of support devices for this challenging patient population,[4,5,24] and the use of objective criteria for the timing of application of MCS is encouraged, as it may improve survival.[25] In general, the guiding principles for success in MCS include appropriate patient selection, meticulous technical deployment, and diligent management in the cardiac intensive care unit with a multidisciplinary shock team.[5,24] Patients with COVID-19 and CS present unique challenges to an already complex and critically ill patient population, the anticipation of which can help guide the clinician caring for these patients on MCS.

MECHANICAL CIRCULATORY SUPPORT IN COVID-19: OUTCOMES AND CONSIDERATIONS
Circulatory Support

For COVID-19 patients suffering from myocardial infarction, the limited data available suggest a significantly increased mortality rate, especially for those who require some type of MCS. Data from the NACMI registry showed an almost 60% mortality rate in COVID-19–positive STEMI patients who required MCS, compared with a 30% mortality rate in non-COVID STEMI patients on MCS.[26] In this registry, 13% of COVID-19–positive STEMI patients received MCS, similar to rates seen in the non-COVID-19 population, highlighting the significant increase in mortality that a concomitant COVID-19 infection conferred. Within the COVID-19 group, the most prevalent type of MCS was the IABP (62%), followed by Impella (28%) and ECMO (7%). Data for or against a particular MCS strategy is limited by the lack of high-quality evidence in the CS patient population. Although the IABP remains commonly used for CS patients requiring MCS, longitudinal data have confirmed that these devices do not confer a mortality benefit.[27] Percutaneous left ventricular assist devices such as the Impella have shown some improvement in small clinical trials and registry data, although the evidence remains mixed and definitive research is ongoing.[28] For these strategies in COVID-19 patients, the data are even more scarce. Case reports exist of using IABPs or Impellas to support hemodynamics in patients with COVID-19 and CS, with mixed outcomes.[12,29]

VA ECMO for cardiovascular collapse in the COVID-19 population represents the maximal level of support possible and brings with it a high rate of morbidity and mortality—so high, perhaps, that many centers may not offer it in this patient population. Indeed, the Extracorporeal Life Support Organization (ELSO) cautions centers about performing extracorporeal cardiopulmonary resuscitation (defined as the insertion of VA ECMO in patients who are pericardiac arrest) on patients with COVID-19, especially in less experienced centers, because of both the technical complexity of the procedure and the risk of cross-contamination to staff.[30]

For COVID-19 patients requiring cardiac support with VA ECMO, ELSO guidelines suggest judicious patient selection in a multidisciplinary manner. Like all MCS, VA ECMO is not a definitive treatment, but is instead a bridge to a destination, be it recovery, durable ventricular assist device, or transplant. Patients with multisystem organ failure, significant medical comorbidities, or advanced age likely do not benefit from VA ECMO support, even without the added complication of an active COVID-19 infection.[31] Some presentations of CS portend slightly better prognoses (eg, myocarditis), whereas other patients with concomitant distributive or inflammatory shock will likely have worse outcomes. On the whole, the decision to place any patient—especially those with an active

COVID-19 infection—on VA ECMO should be a thoughtful, team-based decision with a clear exit strategy in mind. Some centers describe an algorithmic approach to MCS in these patients, favoring the initiation of V-A-V ECMO in COVID-19 patients with CS and refractory hypoxemia,[29] although survival rates of this strategy are unknown.

Overall, data on outcomes for patients with COVID-19 requiring VA ECMO for CS are extremely limited.[31] A large retrospective review of ELSO data found that VA ECMO represents a significant minority of all COVID-19 ECMO cases, perhaps as low as 4%, but is associated with a significantly higher in-hospital mortality rate compared with COVID-19 patients on VV ECMO.[32] ELSO itself does not directly report COVID-19 VA ECMO survival on its public dashboard, but at the time of publication, the survival rate to discharge in the COVID-19 non-ARDS adult cohort is less than 10%.[33] The EuroELSO survey of adult COVID-19 patients in Europe demonstrates a significant decline in the application of VA ECMO in this patient population as the pandemic has progressed, with VA ECMO representing 9% of all COVID-19 ECMO cases at the onset of the pandemic, but falling to an average of 4% during the fourth wave.[34]

The remainder of our current data is limited to case series and case reports, most of which report significant mortality rates for VA ECMO in COVID-19, far above prepandemic benchmarks.[35] Although more information is certainly needed about this patient population to guide thoughtful application and patient selection, it can be said that mortality rates for COVID-19 patients requiring any degree of MCS are high, and VA ECMO portends an even higher risk of death. Centers and clinicians who choose to pursue any MCS strategy in COVID-19 patients must do so thoughtfully and selectively, understanding the inherent risks and resources required.

Respiratory Support

For patients with severe acute respiratory distress syndrome (ARDS), be it from COVID-19 or another pulmonary insult, VV ECMO remains a salvage and off-label therapy for lung rescue for certain patient populations. The largest randomized controlled trial investigating VV ECMO for severe ARDS, conducted in the pre-COVID-19 era, was technically a negative trial,[36] although meta-analyses have shown some benefit for VV ECMO for refractory ARDS,[32] and subsequently its use in the adult population has increased significantly over the past 20 years. Although there are no universal guidelines, inclusion criteria from the EOILA trial are often used to evaluate VV ECMO candidacy, and include a $Pa_{O_2}:Fi_{O_2}$ ratio of less than 50 mm Hg despite maximal medical therapy for ARDS or a refractory respiratory acidosis.[36] According to the ELSO registry, ARDS patients requiring VV ECMO in 2018 had an overall survival rate of approximately 62%.[37] It is understandable, then, that VV ECMO posed an attractive option for patients with severe COVID-19–related ARDS at the beginning of the pandemic, when initial data suggested an up to 97% 28-day mortality rate for intubated COVID-19 patients.[38] After the first wave, some initial registry data were encouraging: mortality for COVID-19 patients on VV ECMO was less than 40%, which was in line with prepandemic outcomes.[32] However, much of that initial enthusiasm has been since tempered, as subsequent waves of the pandemic have shown diminishing returns from the application of VV ECMO in this patient population. Registry data revealed a significant increase in mortality as the pandemic has progressed: after May 2020, mortality for this cohort rose above 50%.[39] Although the underlying reasons for this decline remain somewhat unclear, the available evidence does suggest some possible etiologies.

As the pandemic progressed, more centers with less overall ECMO experience began offering VV ECMO to COVID-19 patients. Registry data did show that hospitals with less ECMO experience witnessed higher mortality rates than more experienced ECMO centers,[39] potentially underscoring the challenges of expanding a complex technology to centers with less volume or training. A recent observational study showed an increased risk of mortality for patients cannulated at a nonspecialized center.[40] In addition, improved medical management of COVID-19 patients, including the use of systemic steroids and antiviral agents together with improved noninvasive oxygenation and ventilation strategies,[41–43] may have led to a sicker, "nonresponder" phenotype of patients being referred for VV ECMO. Although previous VV ECMO studies for ARDS patients had clear inclusion criteria—including, for example, less than 7 days of invasive ventilation[36]—the COVID-19 pandemic challenged these norms. As more patients languished on noninvasive ventilation for weeks before intubation, identifying a cohort of patients who would benefit from VV ECMO has become increasingly challenging. Although avoiding ventilator-induced lung injury is a well-known concept in modern ARDS management and remains the ultimate goal of the "lung rest" afforded by VV ECMO,[44] non–ventilator-associated barotrauma and patient-induced lung injury are not as clearly defined and are ongoing areas of research.[45] Although some treatment strategies may decrease the number of COVID-19 patients who progress to severe ARDS, there is a real risk of delaying recognition of the cohort of patients who are actively declining with respect to their respiratory disease and are within the window to benefit from VV ECMO. Patients who presented with evidence of barotrauma before intubation, for example, posed challenges to ECMO teams—would these patients receive any benefit from the "lung rest" of VV ECMO?—, and many centers adopted more restrictive VV ECMO inclusion criteria for COVID-19 patients as the pandemic progressed.[40] Some centers applied a more aggressive strategy of earlier VV ECMO cannulation: one small retrospective study showed lower mortality rates with early VV ECMO use, and a significantly lower mortality rate of 25% for patients who were cannulated before intubation.[46]

However, VV ECMO remains a technically challenging and personnel-intensive limited resource, with significant risks associated with its use, and clear guidelines on how and when to apply this technology to COVID-19 patients remain unclear.[47] Unfortunately, most of the data on VV ECMO during COVID-19 comes from retrospective studies, case series, and international registries, which lack control groups or randomization, and are often subject to reporting bias. The heterogeneity between survivors and nonsurvivors of ARDS following COVID-19 is becoming clearer, but the scientific community continues to lack the ability to reliably predict which patients may benefit from VV ECMO and in what manner that technology should be applied. As the body of evidence in this patient population grows, institutions must remain flexible about applying clear inclusion criteria for these patients which reflect best practices for VV ECMO but also take into consideration the resources of the institution or region, as this can significantly impact mortality rates as well.[40] Further studies are needed to focus on defining and identifying severe ARDS phenotypes to better assess the efficacy of such a resource-intensive technology as VV ECMO.

SUMMARY

The COVID-19 pandemic has significantly impacted almost all aspects of modern health care, including increased mortality rates for classically described disease processes. For patients with underlying cardiac disease, concomitant COVID-19 infection significantly increases morbidity and mortality and may precipitate conditions such as CS. Although randomized controlled data are sorely lacking, retrospective evidence shows that patients with COVID-19 and CS are sicker and are more likely to die compared with traditional controls. Similarly, COVID-19 patients with isolated respiratory failure and ARDS seem to have increased challenges compared with historical outcomes. The application of MCS to this patient population remains technically complex and resource intensive, carrying with it a significant mortality rate. Although the scientific community awaits more evidence-based practice guidelines for MCS for COVID-19 patients, the necessity of a thoughtful, multidisciplinary team approach to these challenging cases at high-volume, experienced centers remains of the utmost importance.

DISCLOSURE

All authors have nothing to disclose.

REFERENCES

1. Jentzer JC, et al. Cardiogenic shock classification to predict mortality in the cardiac intensive care Unit. J Am Coll Cardiol 2019;74(17):2117–28.
2. Jollis JG, et al. Impact of Regionalization of ST-segment-elevation myocardial infarction care on treatment times and outcomes for Emergency medical Services-Transported patients presenting to hospitals with percutaneous coronary Intervention: Mission: Lifeline Accelerator-2. Circulation 2018; 137(4):376–87.
3. Kolte D, et al. Trends in incidence, management, and outcomes of cardiogenic shock complicating ST-elevation myocardial infarction in the United States. J Am Heart Assoc 2014;3(1):e000590.
4. Smith T, Gorder K. *Ch 21: Regionalization and Protocolization of the Treatment of cardiogenic Shock and Need for mechanical circulatory support devices*. In: Abraham J, Parrillo J, editors. M*echanical circulatory support Devices in the intensive care Unit: Post-Implant Care and management*. Society of Critical Care Medicine; 2021.
5. Henry TD, et al. Invasive management of acute myocardial infarction complicated by cardiogenic shock: a scientific statement from the American Heart association. Circulation 2021;143(15): e815–29.
6. Papolos AI, et al. Management and outcomes of cardiogenic shock in cardiac ICUs with versus without shock teams. J Am Coll Cardiol 2021; 78(13):1309–17.
7. Garan AR, et al. Complete hemodynamic Profiling with pulmonary artery catheters in cardiogenic shock is associated with lower in-hospital mortality. JACC Heart Fail 2020;8(11):903–13.

8. Grasselli G, et al. Pathophysiology of COVID-19-associated acute respiratory distress syndrome: a multicentre prospective observational study. Lancet Respir Med 2020;8(12):1201–8.

9. Mountantonakis SE, et al. Increased Inpatient mortality for cardiovascular patients during the first wave of the COVID-19 Epidemic in New York. J Am Heart Assoc 2021;10(16):e020255.

10. Babapoor-Farrokhran S, et al. Myocardial injury and COVID-19: possible mechanisms. Life Sci 2020;253: 117723.

11. Rusu I, Turlacu M, Micheu MM. Acute myocardial injury in patients with COVID-19: possible mechanisms and clinical implications. World J Clin Cases 2022;10(3):762–76.

12. Valchanov K, et al. COVID-19 patient with coronary thrombosis supported with ECMO and Impella 5.0 ventricular assist device: a case report. Eur Heart J Case Rep 2020;4(6):1–6.

13. Patone M, Mei XW, Handunnetthi L, et al. Risks of myocarditis, pericarditis, and cardiac arrhythmias associated with COVID-19 vaccination or SARS-CoV-2 infection. Nat Med 2022;28:410–22.

14. Purdy A, et al. Myocarditis in COVID-19 presenting with cardiogenic shock: a case series. Eur Heart J Case Rep 2021;5(2):ytab028.

15. Murk W, et al. Diagnosis-wide analysis of COVID-19 complications: an exposure-crossover study. CMAJ 2021;193(1):E10–8.

16. Szekely Y, et al. Spectrum of cardiac manifestations in COVID-19: a systematic Echocardiographic study. Circulation 2020;142(4):342–53.

17. Daniels CJ, et al. Prevalence of clinical and Subclinical myocarditis in Competitive Athletes with recent SARS-CoV-2 infection: results from the Big ten COVID-19 cardiac registry. JAMA Cardiol 2021; 6(9):1078–87.

18. Kite TA, et al. International prospective registry of acute coronary syndromes in patients with COVID-19. J Am Coll Cardiol 2021;77(20): 2466–76.

19. Garcia S, et al. Initial Findings from the North American COVID-19 myocardial infarction registry. J Am Coll Cardiol 2021;77(16):1994–2003.

20. Varshney AS, et al. Epidemiology of cardiogenic shock in Hospitalized adults with COVID-19: a report from the American Heart association COVID-19 cardiovascular disease registry. Circ Heart Fail 2021; 14(12):e008477.

21. Thiele H, et al. Intra-aortic balloon counterpulsation in acute myocardial infarction complicated by cardiogenic shock (IABP-SHOCK II): final 12 month results of a randomised, open-label trial. Lancet 2013;382(9905):1638–45.

22. Baran DA, et al. SCAI clinical expert consensus statement on the classification of cardiogenic shock: this document was endorsed by the American College of Cardiology (ACC), the American Heart association (AHA), the Society of critical care medicine (SCCM), and the Society of Thoracic Surgeons (STS) in April 2019. Catheter Cardiovasc Interv 2019;94(1):29–37.

23. Fincke R, et al. Cardiac power is the strongest hemodynamic correlate of mortality in cardiogenic shock: a report from the SHOCK trial registry. J Am Coll Cardiol 2004;44(2):340–8.

24. van Diepen S, et al. Contemporary management of cardiogenic shock: a scientific statement from the American Heart association. Circulation 2017; 136(16):e232–68.

25. Smith T, G K, Rudick S, et al. Implementing an Algorithm for mechanical support in cardiogenic shock improves survival. J Heart Lung Transplant 2021; 40(4):S183.

26. Guddeti RSC, Jauhar R, Henry T, et al. Mechanical circulatory support in COVID-19 patients presenting with myocardial infarction: Insight from the North American COVID-19 myocardial infarction registry. Submitted. JACC Cardiovasc Interv 2022.

27. Thiele H, Zeymer U, Thelemann N, et al. Intraaortic Balloon Pump in Cardiogenic Shock Complicating Acute Myocardial Infarction. Circulation 2019; 139(3):395–403.

28. Zeymer U, et al. Acute Cardiovascular Care Association position statement for the diagnosis and treatment of patients with acute myocardial infarction complicated by cardiogenic shock: a document of the Acute Cardiovascular Care Association of the European Society of Cardiology. Eur Heart J Acute Cardiovasc Care 2020;9(2):183–97.

29. Ranard LS, et al. Approach to acute cardiovascular complications in COVID-19 infection. Circ Heart Fail 2020;13(7):e007220.

30. Bartlett RH, et al. Initial ELSO guidance document: ECMO for COVID-19 patients with severe cardiopulmonary failure. ASAIO J 2020;66(5):472–4.

31. Chow J, et al. Cardiovascular collapse in COVID-19 infection: the Role of Venoarterial extracorporeal membrane oxygenation (VA-ECMO). CJC Open 2020;2(4):273–7.

32. Barbaro RP, et al. Extracorporeal membrane oxygenation support in COVID-19: an international cohort study of the Extracorporeal Life Support Organization registry. Lancet 2020;396(10257):1071–8.

33. Registry dashboard of ECMO-supported COVID-19 patient data. 2/18/22]. Available at: www.elso.org/Registry/FullCOVID-19RegistryDashboard.aspx.

34. EuroELSO Survey on ECMO use in adult COVID-19 patients in Europe. 2/18/22]. Available at: www.euroelso.net/covid-19/covid-19-survey/.

35. Sromicki J, et al. ECMO therapy in COVID-19: an experience from Zurich. J Card Surg 2021;36(5): 1707–12.

36. Combes A, et al. Extracorporeal membrane oxygenation for severe acute respiratory distress syndrome. N Engl J Med 2018;378(21):1965–75.

37. Extracorporeal Life Support Organization. ECLS registry report international summary. 2019. Available at: https://www.elso.org/Portals/0/Files/Reports/2019/International%20Summary%20January%202019.pdf. Accessed date 28 February 2022.

38. Wang Y, et al. Clinical Course and outcomes of 344 intensive care patients with COVID-19. Am J Respir Crit Care Med 2020;201(11):1430–4.

39. Barbaro RP, et al. Extracorporeal membrane oxygenation for COVID-19: evolving outcomes from the international extracorporeal Life support Organization registry. Lancet 2021;398(10307):1230–8.

40. Gannon WD, Stokes JW, Francois SA, et al. Association between availability of ECMO and mortality in COVID-19 patients eligible for ECMO: a natural experiment. Am J Respir Crit Care Med 2022. Available at: https://pubmed.ncbi.nlm.nih.gov/35212255/.

41. Group RC, et al. Dexamethasone in hospitalized patients with covid-19. N Engl J Med 2021;384(8):693–704.

42. Beigel JH, et al. Remdesivir for the treatment of Covid-19 - final report. N Engl J Med 2020;383(19):1813–26.

43. Papoutsi E, et al. Effect of timing of intubation on clinical outcomes of critically ill patients with COVID-19: a systematic review and meta-analysis of non-randomized cohort studies. Crit Care 2021;25(1):121.

44. Slutsky AS, Ranieri VM. Ventilator-induced lung injury. N Engl J Med 2014;370(10):980.

45. Grieco DL, et al. Non-invasive ventilatory support and high-flow nasal oxygen as first-line treatment of acute hypoxemic respiratory failure and ARDS. Intensive Care Med 2021;47(8):851–66.

46. Kunavarapu C, et al. Clinical outcomes of severe COVID-19 patients receiving early VV-ECMO and the impact of pre-ECMO ventilator use. Int J Artif Organs 2021;44(11):861–7.

47. Badulak J, et al. Extracorporeal membrane oxygenation for COVID-19: Updated 2021 guidelines from the extracorporeal Life support Organization. ASAIO J 2021;67(5):485–95.

Extracardiac Prothrombotic Effects of COVID-19

Rohan Kankaria, BS[a], Cristina Sanina, MD[a,b], Mohamed Gabr, MD[a,b],
Jose Wiley, MD, MPH[a,b], Anna E. Bortnick, MD, PhD, MSc[a,b,c],*

KEYWORDS

- SARS-CoV-2 • COVID-19 • Thrombosis • Stroke • Deep vein thrombosis • Pulmonary embolism
- Myocardial infarction

KEY POINTS

- Microvascular thrombosis has macrovascular effects, leading to gross organ dysfunction in COVID-19 infection.
- There is a greater incidence of macrovascular complications such as venous thrombosis, pulmonary embolism (PE), myocardial infarction (MI), and stroke in individuals affected by COVID-19.
- Anticoagulation with unfractionated and low-molecular-weight heparin (LMWH) may be of benefit to reducing thrombosis if started early in the course of COVID-19 illness.
- Prevention of severe COVID-19 illness is important to avoid thrombotic complications, morbidity, and mortality.

INTRODUCTION

The COVID-19 pandemic has had devastating effects on global health, with greater than 220 million cases and greater than 4 million deaths since January 2020 reported to the World Health Organization.[1,2] Highly transmissible variants risk further spread. In addition to acute respiratory failure, COVID-19 has been linked to arterial and venous thrombosis, especially in those with severe disease.[3] In this review, we summarize data on COVID-19 thrombotic complications (**Central Figure**), delineating the micro- and macrovascular complications that can lead to acute and chronic organ dysfunction and treatment protocols that could lessen the burden of thrombosis.

MECHANISM OF THROMBOSIS IN COVID-19 ILLNESS

Viral pulmonary diseases elaborate inflammatory cytokines which have prothrombotic effects in the vasculature of critically ill patients.[4] SARS-CoV-2, the virus causing COVID-19 illness, invades endothelial cells causing local complement activation and inflammation which leads to microvascular thrombosis.[5–7] Amplification of inflammatory and microvascular insult eventually leads to widespread macrovascular thrombotic injury. Patients with COVID-19 experience both venous and arterial thrombosis.

MICROVASCULAR THROMBOSIS IN COVID-19

Widespread microthrombosis affecting various organ systems is a potential mechanism for long-term sequelae after recovery from COVID-19 which requires investigation. Patients with COVID-19 seem to experience subclinical microvascular thrombosis before developing gross venous or arterial events.[5] One study examining 13 critically ill patients with COVID-19 on mechanical ventilation detected sublingual microthrombi

This article originally appeared in Cardiology Clinics, Volume 40, Issue 3, August 2022.
Funding: AEB is supported, in part, by grant K23HL146982 from the National Heart, Lung, and Blood Institute.
[a] Albert Einstein College of Medicine, Montefiore Medical Center, 1300 Morris Park Avenue, Bronx, NY 10461, USA; [b] Department of Medicine, Division of Cardiology, Montefiore Medical Center, 111 E 210th Street, Bronx, NY 10467 USA; [c] Division of Geriatrics, Montefiore Medical Center, 111 E 210th Street, Bronx, NY 10467 USA
* Corresponding author. Jack D. Weiler Hospital, 1825 Eastchester Road, Suite 2S-46, Bronx, NY 10461.
E-mail address: abortnic@montefiore.org

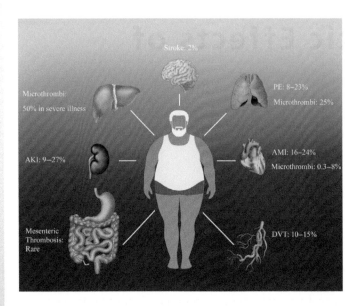

Central Figure. COVID-19 infection predisposes patients to microvascular and macrovascular thrombotic injuries at a higher incidence than the general population. Estimates rounded up. (Compiled from references[10,11,13,20,21,25–27,29–37,43–45,55]. Courtesy of T Harris, Bronx, New York.)

using capillaroscopy, despite none of the patients meeting criteria for diffuse intravascular coagulation.[8] Platelet-rich thrombi have been detected in the pulmonary, renal, cardiac, and hepatic microvasculature, with histopathology indicating increased presence megakaryocytes, a finding suggestive of a cytokine-mediated thrombosis.[9]

PULMONARY MICROVASCULAR THROMBI

Pulmonary injury in patients with COVID-19 may extend beyond diffuse alveolar disease from acute respiratory distress syndrome. Autopsy reports, though limited, demonstrate extensive complement deposition and diffuse microthrombi predominantly in the septal capillaries.[7,9,10] In a case series of 31 patients with COVID-19, 25% of those with elevated D-dimer levels (>1000 ng/mL) had pulmonary perfusion deficits on computed tomography angiography, but only 2 were noted to have gross pulmonary embolism (PE).[10] Patients with perfusion deficits had higher intensive care unit (ICU) admission rates (37.5% vs 4.3%, $P = .043$), higher body mass indices (BMI) (28.85 vs 25.94 $P = .040$), and higher likelihood of severe disease (50% vs 4.3%, $P = .01$) when compared with patients without perfusion deficits.[10]

RENAL MICROVASCULAR THROMBI

The incidence of acute kidney injury (AKI) in patients with COVID-19 is high, from 9% to 27% in retrospective studies, and similar to patients who have other pneumonias.[11–13] Many factors contribute to AKI, but findings from biopsy studies suggest that it is compounded by microvascular

thrombosis. Autopsies from 6 patients showed widespread acute tubular necrosis and glomerular capillary damage from complement activity.[11] Viral inclusions were found in kidney cells supporting direct infection as a mechanism of localized cell death and inflammatory response. Renal perfusion deficits have been observed on imaging, as well.[10] Renal biopsy studies, though limited, demonstrate thrombotic microangiopathy, complement deposition in the mesangial space, fibrin thrombi in the glomeruli, and cortical necrosis in patients with severe AKI.[14,15] Hypercoagulability, defined as a low ADMATS13/VWF antigen ratio, was strongly associated with worsened AKI and severe illness, further supporting renal microthrombosis as a contributory factor to the high incidence of AKI in patients with COVID-19.[16]

DERMATOLOGIC AND OPHTHALMOLOGIC MICROVASCULAR THROMBI

There have been multiple case reports of dermatologic and ophthalmologic microvascular thrombosis.[7,17–19] Patients with pulmonary hemorrhage on autopsy were also found to have complement deposition in the dermal microvasculature.[7] Inflammation of the dermal microvasculature (chilblains) has been reported.[17] Interestingly, complement deposition in skin has also been documented from patients with COVID-19 who did not exhibit pulmonary deficits or obvious skin findings.[7]

There is a singular report of retinal vasculitis in a child, as well as an autopsy series demonstrating ocular endothelial cell damage and fibrin microvascular thrombi in severe COVID-19 illness.[17,18] However, a larger retrospective cohort study found no significant difference when comparing patients with COVID-19 and controls for vascular perfusion in the superficial or deep vascular plexus of the eye, suggesting that it is possible that microthrombi may dissipate with the resolution of disease or that the eye may be spared in many instances.[19]

MYOCARDIAL MICROVASCULAR THROMBI

COVID-19 illness has been associated with myocardial infarction (MI), myocarditis, and cardiomyopathy (reviewed in Kite and colleagues' article, "The Direct and Indirect Effects of COVID-19 on Acute Coronary Syndromes," in this issue). The incidence of MI in patients with COVID-19 has been estimated to range from 0.33% to 8%.[20,21] COVID-19-associated ST-elevation myocardial infarction (STEMI) has been well described and is associated with higher mortality compared with STEMI in patients without COVID-19 infection.[22] However, there are few studies analyzing the extent of microvascular injury in the myocardium. Autopsies of 7 patients showed fibrin microthrombi and megakaryocytes within the myocardial microvasculature in all patients and 2 had macrovascular myocardial venous thrombosis.[9] In a larger, multi-center autopsy study of 21 patients, 4 had fibrin and platelet microthrombi (PMT) in the myocardial microvasculature and 3 had fibrin and PMT in the endocardial microvasculature.[23] These results suggest that patients with severe COVID-19 infection are predisposed to developing myocardial microthrombi. Further studies are necessary to understand the long-term clinical effects on cardiac function.

HEPATIC MICROVASCULAR THROMBI

COVID-19 illness is associated with acute liver injury. Proposed mechanisms of injury are systemic inflammation, hepatic ischemia, drug toxicity, and hepatic microthrombi, which have been seen on autopsy.[9,24] A series of postmortem liver biopsies in patients with COVID-19, without preexisting liver disease or clinical signs of hepatic failure, found that greater than 50% had sinusoidal microthrombi and those individuals had 10-fold higher liver enzyme levels than those who did not have microthrombi.[25] Liver involvement in severe COVID-19 infection was confirmed in a second autopsy series demonstrating hepatic steatosis and elevated megakaryocytes in hepatic sinusoids, which were associated with systemically elevated D-dimer and liver enzyme levels in those individuals.[26]

Importantly, 2 types of microthrombi have been described in hepatic sinusoids: sinusoidal erythrocyte aggregation (SEA) and PMT. PMT thrombosis was associated with significant steatosis as compared with patients with COVID-19 without sinusoidal microthrombosis (79% vs 35%, $P = .02$).[25] Both PMT and SEA thrombosis were associated with significant neutrophil accumulation in the hepatic sinusoids, illustrating the inflammatory component of microthrombotic injury. Compared with SEA, patients with PMT thrombosis were found to have increased incidence of liver injury.[25]

Conversely, a third large autopsy series found minimal microthrombi, with 50% having mild hepatitis and 75% with macrovesicular steatosis. Hepatic vascular findings were limited to scarce nondiffuse vascular abnormalities with 6 patients showing signs of veno-occlusive disease and 5 patients showing signs of arteriolar muscular hyperplasia.[27] Of note, in all 3 autopsy studies, steatosis was not associated with obesity or diabetes, suggesting that hepatic steatosis in these decedents of COVID-19 was not secondary to nonalcoholic fatty liver disease, but more likely a consequence of inflammation.[25]

MACROVASCULAR THROMBOSIS IN COVID-19

The mechanism of macrovascular thrombosis seems to be an extension of the proposed mechanisms delineating microvascular thrombosis. Pro-inflammatory mediated cytokine release and direct endothelial damage activate the coagulation cascade leading to widespread macrovascular thrombosis, including PE, deep vein thrombosis (DVT), stroke, and MI.[28]

PULMONARY EMBOLISM

COVID-19 has been associated with an increased incidence of PE ranging from 8.3% to 23%, depending on the severity of illness, based on retrospective studies.[29–31] In comparison, the incidence of any venous thrombosis in the general population is 0.1%.[32] There is conflicting evidence that obesity predisposes to developing PE in the context of COVID-19 and it may depend on the severity of illness. Male sex and concomitant cardiovascular disease (CVD) are potentially predisposing factors, as well.[31] Multiple studies indicate that patients with PE have higher D-dimer levels when compared with patients with COVID-19 without PE, suggesting that D-dimer levels can be used for diagnostics, prognostic purposes, and risk stratification.[29–31]

In a study of moderate COVID-19, there was a lower incidence of PE (8.3%) and neither obesity nor diabetes was predisposing factors.[30] Patients who were treated with anticoagulation, either prophylactic or therapeutic dose, low-molecular-weight heparin (LMWH) or subcutaneous unfractionated heparin (UFH) before or during hospitalization, had a significantly lower odds for developing PE.[30] Importantly, PE was more likely to develop in patients with delayed hospitalization.[30] Interestingly, in a study of all-comers on statins predating mild, moderate or severe COVID-19 illness, treatment resulted in a significantly lower odds ratio (OR) of PE; OR: 0.4 [95%, confidence interval (CI): 0.23–0.75].[29] Thus, anticoagulation, statins, and modulating the intensity of the inflammatory response to COVID-19 may be helpful in avoiding PE in hospitalized individuals.

VENOUS THROMBOEMBOLISM AND ARTERIAL THROMBOEMBOLIC COMPLICATIONS

Multi-center inpatient studies show a 10% to 14.7% incidence of venous thromboembolism in COVID-19 illness compared with 0.1% of the general population, but up to as high as 45.4% in ICU-level patients.[32–35] Many develop asymptomatic DVT. Some centers only screened symptomatic patients; thus, the incidence is likely underreported in those studies. Like PE, patients with COVID-19 with DVT had higher D-dimer levels.[34–36] There were no differences in baseline sex, age, or BMI of patients with COVID-19 who developed DVT as compared with those who did not, in limited studies.[34–36] Additionally, DVT was linked to worse multi-system organ function and breakthrough from prophylactic anticoagulation.

A large, single-center, retrospective study of 362 patients found an incidence of total venous and arterial thromboembolic events of 7.7%, but this number may be underestimated as there was no surveillance of asymptomatic patients.[36] Most of those diagnosed with DVT also had concomitant PE; nonsurvivors had higher D-dimer levels.[36]

A prospective study of 156 COVID-19 positive inpatients evaluated the incidence of asymptomatic DVT. Patients received standard DVT prophylaxis of enoxaparin 40 mg per day or bemiparin 3500 IU per day. Of the 156 surveilled, 23 patients (14.7%) developed DVT with the majority (22/23) developing distal DVT. Patients who developed DVT had higher average D-dimer levels than those without (4527 vs 2050 ng/mL, $P < .001$).[35] There was no significant difference in obesity, sex, or age in patients who developed DVT versus those who did not.[35]

The incidence of DVT seems higher in critically ill patients with COVID-19.[34] In a retrospective, single-center analysis of 88 ICU patients receiving thromboprophylaxis with LMWH, 40 developed DVT (45.4%).[34] In this study, DVT was not associated with BMI, age, sex, and platelet counts, but was associated with elevated sequential organ failure assessment (SOFA) scores (6 vs 4, $P < .001$), elevated D-dimer levels (6.4 vs 3.1 mg/L, $P < .02$), hypoalbuminemia (28.81 vs 32.39 g/L, $P < .001$) and longer duration of illness (34 vs 20 days, $P = .007$). Anatomically, most DVTs were distal and bilateral.[34] Thus, prophylactic LMWH may be insufficient for the prevention of DVT in the ICU population.

STROKE

The incidence of stroke in COVID-19 infection is approximately 1.7%.[37] By comparison, the risk of stroke in the general population is 0.2%.[38] Studies point to severe COVID-19 infection or underlying cardiovascular risk factors as highly contributory to stroke.[39,40] In comparison to incident DVT and PE, there seems to be a stronger association of underlying CVD risk factors with COVID-19-associated stroke.

Retrospective case-control studies have documented increased stroke in hospitalized COVID-19 patients, and conversely, more frequent COVID-19 infection in those hospitalized with stroke during the time frame of the pandemic. COVID-19 was more often associated with stroke in Black individuals in a larger, multicenter analysis.[39] Black individuals with COVID-19 comprised a greater proportion of stroke cases compared with noninfected Black controls (44.7% vs 19.6%, $P < .0001$).[39] Conversely, White individuals with COVID-19 accounted for a smaller proportion of stroke cases compared with White individuals without COVID-19 (35.9% vs 56.3, $P < .0001$).[39] Patients with hypertension, type 2 diabetes mellitus (T2DM), atrial fibrillation, and congestive heart failure at baseline were more likely to develop stroke. Hospitalized patients with COVID-19-associated stroke had higher mortality rates (19.4% vs 6.2%, $P < .0001$), longer hospital stay, and more frequently had concomitant MI (10.7% vs 4.6%, $P = .003$).[39]

From March to April 2020, COVID-19 was more frequently diagnosed in those with stroke, after adjusting for age, sex, vascular risk factors, and underlying comorbidities.[41] Patients presenting with stroke were infected with COVID-19 46.3% of the time as compared with 18.3% of the time for nonstroke patients (P = .001).[41] Similar data from a single-center retrospective study support the observation that severe COVID-19, hypertension and T2DM are associated with increased incidence of stroke, but in this study, age was a significant factor as well, with all strokes occurring in patients greater than 60 years.[40] Patients with COVID-19 infected stroke have poorer outcomes and prolonged neurologic deficits, with worse neurologic disabilities at discharge and a higher incidence of delirium than stroke patients without COVID-19.[42]

INTESTINAL VASCULAR COMPLICATIONS

Acute mesenteric ischemia and mesenteric venous thrombosis are rare complications of COVID-19, thus, data are limited.[43–45] Clinicians should be vigilant for intestinal thrombotic injury in the correct context. In a case report, one patient presented with mesenteric venous thrombosis after presenting 20 days after the onset of COVID-19 with severe abdominal pain, suggesting prolonged hypercoagulability in some individuals.[45]

PREVENTION AND TREATMENT OF THROMBOSIS IN COVID-19 INFECTION

There is varying evidence on indications, dose, and efficacy of medical therapy for thrombotic complications of COVID-19. Studies suggest the greatest effect in preventing thrombotic injury is with heparins rather than direct oral anticoagulants (DOAC).[46–49] It is important to note that many studies are nonrandomized and focus on macrovascular rather than microvascular thrombosis.

Heparin has been studied in several randomized controlled clinical trials in noncritically and critically ill patients.[46,47] Patients were randomized to either therapeutic doses of UFH or LMWH based on local dosing protocols or standard thromboprophylaxis. In noncritically ill patients, therapeutic heparin increased organ support-free days, defined as the total number of days without respiratory or cardiovascular support, OR: 1.27 (95% CI: 1.03–1.58). Patients on therapeutic heparin were less likely to die (OR: 0.72 95% CI: 0.53–0.98). There was a nonstatistically significant increase in bleeding (OR: 1.8, 95% CI: 0.9–3.74).[46] By comparison, patients with critically ill COVID-19 on therapeutic anticoagulation did not have a significant improvement in organ support-free days or mortality. Thrombosis and risk of major bleeding were similar between treatment assignments.[47] Thus, the optimal window for therapeutic anticoagulation may be early in the course of illness. Accordingly, in a retrospective study looking at the incidence of PE in patients with COVID-19,

non-ICU level COVID-19 individuals on prophylactic anticoagulation were found to have a lower incidence of PE later in the course of their illness.[30]

DOACs have also been studied in patients with COVID-19.[48] In a large randomized control trial, patients were randomized to therapeutic or prophylactic doses.[48] Most received rivaroxaban; however, unstable patients received enoxaparin and were later switched to rivaroxaban once stable, while a minority received UFH. There was no reduction in the duration of hospitalization or supplemental oxygen, DVT, PE, MI, stroke, or death with therapeutic anticoagulation and there were no differences when stratifying for stability. Clinically significant bleeding events were more common in patients receiving therapeutic anticoagulation (8% vs 2%, P = .001).[48]

Another large multicenter retrospective study demonstrated the benefit of anticoagulation with either warfarin or DOACs (dabigatran, rivaroxaban, or apixaban) predating COVID-19, supporting the hypothesis that early anticoagulation is most beneficial in preventing thrombosis during infection.[49] Patients in this study were older, more likely to have hypertension, T2DM, dyslipidemia, and cardiovascular risk factors; a high-risk group for developing prothrombotic complications of COVID-19. Patients who were on therapeutic oral anticoagulation at baseline had less ICU admission, RR 0.45 (95% CI: 0.32–0.62), and lower combined ICU admission and death, RR 0.72 (95% CI: 0.57–0.9), after adjustment. Anticoagulation after hospitalization did not significantly alter ICU admission or death in this observational cohort.[49] However, this finding is contradicted by a retrospective study of hospitalized patients receiving apixaban, enoxaparin, or heparin.[50] Patients on apixaban at prophylactic or therapeutic doses showed lower adjusted odds for death OR: 0.46, (95% CI: 0.30–0.71) and OR: 0.57, (95% CI: 0.38–0.85), respectively, as compared with patients who were not treated. In this study, neither prophylactic nor therapeutic doses of UFH were of benefit. Stratifying by D-dimer levels indicated that patients with low levels of less than 1 μg/mL did not benefit from anticoagulation therapy. However, patients with D-dimer $\geq$ 1 μg/mL had lower mortality on either enoxaparin at prophylactic doses or apixaban at prophylactic or therapeutic doses.[50]

A recent, multicenter, randomized controlled trial studied the use of antiplatelet and anticoagulation therapy in outpatients symptomatic of COVID-19. Patients were randomized into one of the following arms: aspirin 81 mg once daily, apixaban 2.5 mg twice daily (prophylactic dosage), apixaban 5 mg twice daily (therapeutic dosage), or placebo. Patients were excluded if they were previously hospitalized with COVID-19, had other indications for anticoagulation, or had recent major bleeding events.[51] When compared with placebo, treatment with aspirin and apixaban showed no reduction in thrombotic events (DVT, PE, arterial thromboembolism, MI, and stroke). There was an increased risk of minor bleeding in patients receiving therapeutic apixaban with an increased risk difference of 6.9 (95% CI: 1.4–12.9).[51]

Anti-platelet agents, including aspirin, $P2Y_{12}$ inhibitors, and dual antiplatelet therapy (DAPT) do not seem to be beneficial in preventing death or progression of COVID-19 in small retrospective studies.[52,53] A larger, retrospective, multicenter study showed that patients who received aspirin before hospitalization had lower mortality rates, ICU admission, and need for mechanical ventilation.[54] These patients were also more likely to have underlying medical comorbidities such as hypertension, coronary artery disease, and T2DM.

Current therapeutic guidelines to prevent prothrombotic complications of COVID-19 are limited by the lack of sufficient randomized control trials of various anticoagulation and antiplatelet regimens. Limited data from randomized trials suggest that early heparin anticoagulation, before progression to severe COVID -19, may decrease thrombotic complications and death.[30,46,47]

SUMMARY

COVID-19 is associated with multi-organ arterial and venous thrombosis, particularly in individuals who are older, obese, and living with T2DM. Black patients appear more predisposed to COVID-19-associated stroke than White patients. Patients with COVID-19 can develop asymptomatic DVT. Prophylactic LMWH may be insufficient for the prevention of DVT in the ICU population. Anticoagulation with unfractionated and LMWH may be of benefit to reducing thrombosis if started early in the course of COVID-19 illness.

Randomized control trials are necessary to delineate the most effective regimens to prevent and treat thrombotic events from COVID-19 infection. Additional research on long-term consequences of microvascular thrombotic injury and organ dysfunction is required to understand the implications for survivors. Preventing severe infection remains of strategic importance in reducing morbidity and mortality from COVID-19-associated thrombosis.

DISCLOSURE

The authors have no conflicts relating to the published work.

CLINICS CARE POINTS

- Worsening clinical courses such as hypoxia, acute kidney injury (AKI), rising liver enzymes, rising D-dimer levels, or persistent fevers may point to COVID-19 associated thrombosis.
- Prophylactic anticoagulation in mild infection or therapeutic anticoagulation with low molecular weight heparin (LMWH) in moderate or symptomatic disease may prevent major thrombotic events.
- Antifactor Xa activity monitoring may be useful for guiding the titration of therapeutic LMWH in COVID-19 infection.
- Early intervention to slow disease progression may help decrease the risk of associated thrombosis and should be investigated in further research.
- Anticoagulation with unfractionated or LMWH may be insufficient to prevent thrombosis in severe COVID-19 infection. Whether direct thrombin inhibitors are more effective in this context requires investigation, but could be considered in the critically ill.

ACKNOWLEDGMENTS

The authors thank Tatyana A. Harris, Albert Einstein College of Medicine Creative Services, for designing the Central Figure.

REFERENCES

1. Koyama T, Weeraratne D, Snowdon JL, et al. Emergence of Drift variants that may Affect COVID-19 Vaccine Development and Antibody treatment. Pathogens 2020;9(5).
2. Organization WH. WHO coronavirus (COVID-19) Dashboard. 2021. Available at: https://covid19.who.int. Accessed October 1, 2021.
3. Helms J, Tacquard C, Severac F, et al. High risk of thrombosis in patients with severe SARS-CoV-2 infection: a multicenter prospective cohort study. Intensive Care Med 2020;46(6):1089–98.
4. Goeijenbier M, van Wissen M, van de Weg C, et al. Review: Viral infections and mechanisms of thrombosis and bleeding. J Med Virol 2012;84(10):1680–96.
5. Page EM, Ariens RAS. Mechanisms of thrombosis and cardiovascular complications in COVID-19. Thromb Res 2021;200:1–8.
6. Varga Z, Flammer AJ, Steiger P, et al. Endothelial cell infection and endotheliitis in COVID-19. Lancet 2020;395(10234):1417–8.

7. Magro C, Mulvey JJ, Berlin D, et al. Complement associated microvascular injury and thrombosis in the pathogenesis of severe COVID-19 infection: a report of five cases. Transl Res 2020;220:1–13.

8. do Espirito Santo DA, Lemos ACB, Miranda CH. In vivo demonstration of microvascular thrombosis in severe COVID-19. J Thromb Thrombolysis 2020; 50(4):790–4.

9. Rapkiewicz AV, Mai X, Carsons SE, et al. Megakaryocytes and platelet-fibrin thrombi characterize multi-organ thrombosis at autopsy in COVID-19: a case series. EClinicalMedicine 2020;24:100434.

10. Idilman IS, Telli Dizman G, Ardali Duzgun S, et al. Lung and kidney perfusion deficits diagnosed by dual-energy computed tomography in patients with COVID-19-related systemic microangiopathy. Eur Radiol 2021;31(2):1090–9.

11. Diao B, Wang C, Wang R, et al. Human kidney is a target for novel severe acute respiratory syndrome coronavirus 2 infection. Nat Commun 2021;12(1): 2506.

12. Sise ME, Baggett MV, JO Shepard, et al. Case 17-2020: a 68-year-Old man with Covid-19 and acute kidney injury. N Engl J Med 2020;382(22):2147–56.

13. Chen YT, Shao SC, Hsu CK, et al. Incidence of acute kidney injury in COVID-19 infection: a systematic review and meta-analysis. Crit Care 2020;24(1):346.

14. Boudhabhay I, Rabant M, Roumenina LT, et al. Case report: Adult post-COVID-19 Multisystem inflammatory syndrome and thrombotic microangiopathy. Front Immunol 2021;12:680567.

15. Jhaveri KD, Meir LR, Flores Chang BS, et al. Thrombotic microangiopathy in a patient with COVID-19. Kidney Int 2020;98(2):509–12.

16. Henry BM, Benoit SW, de Oliveira MHS, et al. ADAMTS13 activity to von Willebrand factor antigen ratio predicts acute kidney injury in patients with COVID-19: evidence of SARS-CoV-2 induced secondary thrombotic microangiopathy. Int J Lab Hematol 2021;43(Suppl 1):129–36.

17. Quintana-Castanedo L, Feito-Rodriguez M, Fernandez-Alcalde C, et al. Concurrent chilblains and retinal vasculitis in a child with COVID-19. J Eur Acad Dermatol Venereol 2020;34(12):e764–6.

18. Reinhold A, Tzankov A, Matter MS, et al. Ocular pathology and Occasionally detectable Intraocular severe acute respiratory syndrome coronavirus-2 RNA in five fatal coronavirus disease-19 cases. Ophthalmic Res 2021;64(5):785–92.

19. Savastano MC, Gambini G, Cozzupoli GM, et al. Retinal capillary involvement in early post-COVID-19 patients: a healthy controlled study. Graefes Arch Clin Exp Ophthalmol 2021;259(8):2157–65.

20. Modin D, Claggett B, Sindet-Pedersen C, et al. Acute COVID-19 and the incidence of ischemic stroke and acute myocardial infarction. Circulation 2020;142(21):2080–2.

21. Li B, Yang J, Zhao F, et al. Prevalence and impact of cardiovascular metabolic diseases on COVID-19 in China. Clin Res Cardiol 2020;109(5):531–8.

22. Saad M, Kennedy KF, Imran H, et al. Association between COVID-19 Diagnosis and in-hospital mortality in patients hospitalized with ST-Segment elevation myocardial infarction. JAMA 2021;326(19):1940–52.

23. Basso C, Leone O, Rizzo S, et al. Pathological features of COVID-19-associated myocardial injury: a multicentre cardiovascular pathology study. Eur Heart J 2020;41(39):3827–35.

24. Hundt MA, Deng Y, Ciarleglio MM, et al. Abnormal liver Tests in COVID-19: a retrospective observational cohort study of 1,827 patients in a major U.S. Hospital Network. Hepatology 2020;72(4): 1169–76.

25. Kondo R, Kawaguchi N, McConnell MJ, et al. Pathological characteristics of liver sinusoidal thrombosis in COVID-19 patients: a series of 43 cases. Hepatol Res 2021;51(9):1000–6.

26. Zhao CL, Rapkiewicz A, Maghsoodi-Deerwester M, et al. Pathological findings in the postmortem liver of patients with coronavirus disease 2019 (COVID-19). Hum Pathol 2021;109:59–68.

27. Lagana SM, Kudose S, Iuga AC, et al. Hepatic pathology in patients dying of COVID-19: a series of 40 cases including clinical, histologic, and virologic data. Mod Pathol 2020;33(11):2147–55.

28. Kamel MH, Yin W, Zavaro C, et al. Hyperthrombotic Milieu in COVID-19 patients. Cells 2020;9(11).

29. Poyiadji N, Cormier P, Patel PY, et al. Acute pulmonary embolism and COVID-19. Radiology 2020; 297(3):E335–8.

30. Fauvel C, Weizman O, Trimaille A, et al. Pulmonary embolism in COVID-19 patients: a French multicentre cohort study. Eur Heart J 2020;41(32): 3058–68.

31. Faggiano P, Bonelli A, Paris S, et al. Acute pulmonary embolism in COVID-19 disease: Preliminary report on seven patients. Int J Cardiol 2020;313: 129–31.

32. White RH. The epidemiology of venous thromboembolism. Circulation 2003;107(23 Suppl 1):I4–8.

33. Boonyawat K, Chantrathammachart P, Numthavaj P, et al. Incidence of thromboembolism in patients with COVID-19: a systematic review and meta-analysis. Thromb J 2020;18(1):34.

34. Chen S, Zhang D, Zheng T, et al. DVT incidence and risk factors in critically ill patients with COVID-19. J Thromb Thrombolysis 2021;51(1):33–9.

35. Demelo-Rodriguez P, Cervilla-Munoz E, Ordieres-Ortega L, et al. Incidence of asymptomatic deep vein thrombosis in patients with COVID-19 pneumonia and elevated D-dimer levels. Thromb Res 2020;192:23–6.

36. Lodigiani C, Iapichino G, Carenzo L, et al. Venous and arterial thromboembolic complications in

COVID-19 patients admitted to an academic hospital in Milan, Italy. Thromb Res 2020;191:9–14.

37. Siow I, Lee KS, Zhang JJY, et al. Stroke as a neurological complication of COVID-19: a systematic review and meta-analysis of incidence, outcomes and Predictors. J Stroke Cerebrovasc Dis 2021; 30(3):105549.

38. Rosamond WD, Folsom AR, Chambless LE, et al. Stroke incidence and survival among middle-aged adults: 9-year follow-up of the Atherosclerosis Risk in Communities (ARIC) cohort. Stroke 1999;30(4): 736–43.

39. Qureshi AI, Baskett WI, Huang W, et al. Acute ischemic stroke and COVID-19: an analysis of 27 676 patients. Stroke 2021;52(3):905–12.

40. Li Y, Li M, Wang M, et al. Acute cerebrovascular disease following COVID-19: a single center, retrospective, observational study. Stroke Vasc Neurol 2020; 5(3):279–84.

41. Belani P, Schefflein J, Kihira S, et al. COVID-19 is an Independent risk factor for acute ischemic stroke. AJNR Am J Neuroradiol 2020;41(8):1361–4.

42. Benussi A, Pilotto A, Premi E, et al. Clinical characteristics and outcomes of inpatients with neurologic disease and COVID-19 in Brescia, Lombardy, Italy. Neurology 2020;95(7):e910–20.

43. Fan BE, Chang CCR, Teo CHY, et al. COVID-19 Coagulopathy with Superior mesenteric vein thrombosis complicated by an Ischaemic Bowel. Hamostaseologie 2020;40(5):592–3.

44. Singh B, Mechineni A, Kaur P, et al. Acute intestinal ischemia in a patient with COVID-19 infection. Korean J Gastroenterol 2020;76(3):164–6.

45. Aleman W, Cevallos LC. Subacute mesenteric venous thrombosis secondary to COVID-19: a late thrombotic complication in a nonsevere patient. Radiol Case Rep 2021;16(4):899–902.

46. Investigators A, Investigators AC-a, Investigators R-C, et al. Therapeutic anticoagulation with heparin in Noncritically ill patients with Covid-19. N Engl J Med 2021;385(9):790–802.

47. Investigators R-C, Investigators AC-a, Investigators A, et al. Therapeutic anticoagulation with heparin in critically ill patients with Covid-19. N Engl J Med 2021;385(9):777–89.

48. Lopes RD, de Barros ESPGM, Furtado RHM, et al. Therapeutic versus prophylactic anticoagulation for patients admitted to hospital with COVID-19 and elevated D-dimer concentration (ACTION): an open-label, multicentre, randomised, controlled trial. Lancet 2021;397(10291):2253–63.

49. Chocron R, Galand V, Cellier J, et al. Anticoagulation before hospitalization is a potential Protective factor for COVID-19: Insight from a French multicenter cohort study. J Am Heart Assoc 2021;10(8): e018624.

50. Billett HH, Reyes-Gil M, Szymanski J, et al. Anticoagulation in COVID-19: effect of enoxaparin, heparin, and apixaban on mortality. Thromb Haemost 2020; 120(12):1691–9.

51. Connors JM, Brooks MM, Sciurba FC, et al. Effect of antithrombotic therapy on clinical outcomes in outpatients with clinically stable symptomatic COVID-19: the ACTIV-4B randomized clinical trial. JAMA 2021;326(19):1940–52.

52. Russo V, Di Maio M, Attena E, et al. Clinical impact of pre-admission antithrombotic therapy in hospitalized patients with COVID-19: a multicenter observational study. Pharmacol Res 2020;159:104965.

53. Banik JM V, Köhler C, Schmidtmann M. Antiplatelet therapy in patients with Covid-19: a retrospective observational study. Thromb Update 2021;2.

54. Chow JH, Khanna AK, Kethireddy S, et al. Aspirin Use is associated with decreased mechanical ventilation, intensive care Unit admission, and in-hospital mortality in hospitalized patients with coronavirus disease 2019. Anesth Analg 2021;132(4):930–41.

55. Prasitlumkum N, Chokesuwattanaskul R, Thongprayoon C, et al. Incidence of myocardial injury in COVID-19-infected patients: a systematic review and meta-analysis. Diseases (Basel, Switzerland) 2020;8(4).

Impact of COVID-19 on Acute Myocardial Infarction Care

Raviteja R. Guddeti, MD[a], Mehmet Yildiz, MD[b], Keshav R. Nayak, MD[c],
M. Chadi Alraies, MD[d], Laura Davidson, MD[e], Timothy D. Henry, MD[b],
Santiago Garcia, MD[b],*

KEYWORDS

- COVID-19 • Myocardial infarction • STEMI • NSTEMI • Percutaneous coronary intervention
- Fibrinolytic therapy

KEY POINTS

- COVID-19 has negatively impacted the overall care of patients with acute myocardial infarction (MI).
- Globally, there have been significant reductions in hospital admissions, cardiac catheterization laboratory activations, and percutaneous coronary interventions for acute MI, attributed to both patient- and system-related factors.
- Symptom onset to revascularization time increased significantly during the pandemic for both STEMI and NSTEMI, resulting in worse in-hospital outcomes, including all-cause death, cardiogenic shock, and heart failure.
- Although several studies have reported short-term outcomes, future research should focus on examining the long-term effects of the pandemic on this particularly vulnerable patient population.

INTRODUCTION

The coronavirus disease 2019 (COVID-19) outbreak, caused by severe acute respiratory syndrome coronavirus 2 (SARS-CoV-2), was first reported in December 2019 in Wuhan, Hubei Province, China, and has quickly spread to the rest of the world causing a global health crisis. On March 11, 2020, the World Health Organization declared COVID-19 a pandemic. As of November 2021, a total of over 250 million cases have been reported worldwide with over 5 million deaths with a case fatality rate of about 2% (CDC, US Department of Health and Human Services). As of November 2021, the United States has recorded over 46 million confirmed cases of COVID-19 and

over 750,000 deaths. Most patients infected with the SARS-CoV-2 virus are either asymptomatic or minimally symptomatic, which likely underestimates the true prevalence of COVID-19.

This outbreak has quickly overwhelmed health care systems around the world consuming and shifting resources to care for these patients, resulting in deferral or avoidance of care for many non-covid patients, placing those with other health conditions at risk because of limited access to high-quality medical care. Similarly, patients with cardiovascular diseases have been greatly affected as a result. At the beginning of the pandemic, many elective cardiac procedures were canceled to minimize exposure to cardiac

This article originally appeared in Cardiology Clinics, Volume 40, Issue 3, August 2022.
[a] Minneapolis Heart Institute Foundation, Minneapolis, MN 55407, USA; [b] The Christ Hospital Health Network, 2139 Auburn Avenue Suite 424, Cincinnati, OH 45219, USA; [c] Scripps Mercy Hospital, San Diego, CA 92103, USA; [d] DMC Harper University Hospital, Detroit, MI 48201, USA; [e] Northwestern University Feinberg School of Medicine, Chicago, IL 60611, USA
* Corresponding author. The Christ Hospital Health Network, 2139 Auburn Avenue Suite 424, Cincinnati, OH 45219.
E-mail address: santiagogarcia@me.com

Heart Failure Clin 19 (2023) 221–229
https://doi.org/10.1016/j.hfc.2022.08.004

catheterization laboratory personnel and nursing staff with priority given only to the management of ST-segment elevation myocardial infarction (STEMI) and critically ill non–ST-segment elevation myocardial infarction (NSTEMI) patients.

Despite a declining trend in overall incidence, acute myocardial infarction (MI) continues to remain a condition with high morbidity and mortality, with an incidence of 805,000 cases annually.[1] Timely coronary revascularization, achieved by primary percutaneous coronary intervention (PPCI), remains the mainstay of management for acute MI. Data from around the world during the pandemic suggested significantly lower rates of hospitalizations for acute MI, both STEMI and NSTEMI, either due to lower referral rates, patients' hesitancy to seek health care in fear of contracting COVID-19 at the hospitals, or even misdiagnosis.[2–8] We discuss the impact of COVID-19 on the treatment of the important aspects of acute MI.

Impact of COVID-19 on ST-Segment Elevation Myocardial Infarction Care

The COVID-19 pandemic has had a dramatic negative impact on the overall care of STEMI patients (**Fig. 1**).[2–8] The areas most impacted by COVID-19 include:

- Reduction in STEMI activations
- Prolonged symptom-to-first medical contact time
- Prolonged door-to-balloon times
- A shift from PPCI to pharmacologic reperfusion (ie, fibrinolytic therapy)
- Reduction in patients undergoing invasive angiography and PPCI
- Worsening clinical outcomes

ST-segment elevation myocardial infarction activations and hospital admissions

Compared with the prepandemic years, STEMI activations were reduced significantly during the early months of the pandemic. This decrease in STEMI admissions was seen irrespective of age, gender, underlying comorbidities, and geographic region. In the first 3 months of the pandemic between January 2020 and March 2020, a 38% reduction in STEMI activations was noted in the United States compared with the same period the previous year.[2] An expanded and extended analysis of the United States that included 18 large health care systems showed a drop in STEMI activations of about 29%.[9] Interestingly, this drop in STEMI activations affected all geographic regions irrespective of COVID-19 incidence or stay-at-home orders.[9] A similar trend has been reported around the world (**Fig. 2**).[5,8,10] This decrease in STEMI activations coincided with a significant increase in out-of-hospital cardiac arrests, which raised concerns about patients with cardiovascular emergencies foregoing medical care during the pandemic.[11] An increase in mechanical complications of STEMI was also noted.[12]

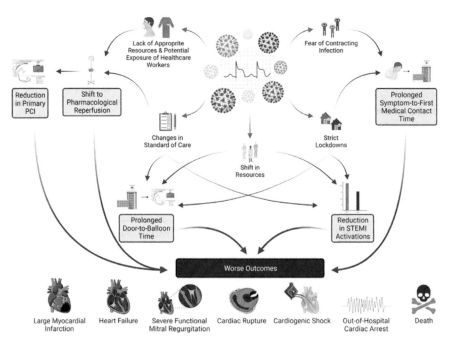

Fig. 1. Impact of COVID-19 on STEMI care (created with BioRender).

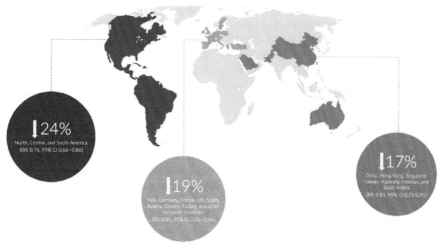

Fig. 2. Reductions in STEMI hospitalizations during the COVID-19 pandemic.[46]

Using data from a National Patient Care database from January 2019 to May 2020, a 23% reduction in weekly STEMI admission rates was reported in the United Kingdom between mid-February and the end of March 2020 compared with the weekly average admissions in 2019.[6] This decline was partially reversed in April and May 2020 to a weekly reduction of 16% by the end of the study period. Similarly, data from Italy showed in March 2020 there was a 26.5% reduction in STEMI admissions compared with the same period the year before.[5] Interestingly, the reduction in admissions was higher among women compared with men (41.2% vs 17.8%), which could represent gender disparity in the management of STEMI during the pandemic.

In addition to the reluctance to seek medical attention by patients out of fear of contracting COVID-19, other potential explanations for the lower rate of STEMI activations during the pandemic include a shift to pharmacologic reperfusion to minimize operator exposure, misdiagnosis of STEMI, and changes in standard of care, including personal protective equipment, emergency medical services (EMSs), rapid testing and hospital beds, and a shift in resources to care for COVID-19 patients. It is unlikely that the reduction in STEMI represents reduced MI incidence related to less physical and work-related stress. The increased numbers of cardiac arrests and late complications of STEMI would suggest otherwise.

Symptom-to-first medical contact and door-to-balloon times

Although evidence suggests that reduced door-to-balloon times have significantly improved outcomes in STEMI,[13,14] patient-related delay (symptom to first medical contact) remains a significant challenge. The total ischemic time, defined as symptom onset to revascularization, is a major determinant of outcomes in STEMI.[15–17] During the current pandemic, this important metric was significantly longer compared with that in the pre-COVID era as demonstrated by Abdelaziz and colleagues.[10] In this study, once the patient presented to the hospital, the door-to-balloon time was similar between the 2 groups, but troponin levels were significantly higher in the COVID era patients (2739 [932–10,480] ng/L vs 1245 [327–2789] ng/L), demonstrating the probable consequences of delayed presentation.

In Italy, De Rosa and colleagues[5] reported a 39.2% increase in symptom-to-coronary angiography time and a 31.5% increase in time from first medical contact to coronary revascularization, which signifies a substantial increase in both patient- and system-related delays. Analysis from the European International Study on Acute Coronary Syndromes-STEMI (ISACS-STEMI) COVID-19 registry demonstrated that the total ischemic time was significantly longer during the pandemic (181 [120–301] min in 2019 vs 200 [127–357] min in 2020; $P = .004$) as was the door-to-balloon time (34 [21–36] min in 2019 vs 36 [24–60] min in 2020; $P = .007$).[18] Delayed presentations beyond 12 hours of ischemic time were also more common during the pandemic (9.1% in 2019 vs 11.7% in 2020; $P < .001$).

The prospective Magnetic Resonance Imaging in Acute ST-Elevation Myocardial Infarction (MARINA-STEMI) evaluated STEMI patients with cardiac magnetic resonance imaging (cMRI) during times of public health restrictions versus no restrictions and provided a mechanistic link between patient delays and poor outcomes. MARINA-STEMI revealed that patients treated during lockdowns had larger infarct sizes (22 [IQR 12–29]% vs 14 [IQR 6–23]%, $P < .01$), more microvascular obstruction (77% vs 52%, $P < .01$) and a higher rate of intramyocardial hemorrhage (56% vs 34%, $P = .02$).[19]

Both patient- and system-related factors appear to have contributed to delay in symptom-to-first medical contact and door-to-balloon times during the pandemic, which limits the substantial benefit provided by primary PCI in STEMI. Fear of contracting COVID-19 infection at the hospital or the physician's office often seems to have led patients to delay seeking appropriate care for chest pain. Early in the pandemic, health care systems were stressed, which impacted the timely management of STEMI patients. Multiple countries implemented strict lockdowns to prevent the spread of COVID-19 with both hospital and EMSs redirected to critically ill COVID-19 patients. Longer EMS response times and shortages of experienced EMS personnel contributed to delays in cardiac catheterization laboratory activations from the field. These differences were more pronounced in countries that entered the pandemic with limited health care resources in infrastructure and personnel. In a systematic review, Chew and colleagues[20] demonstrated that low-income countries reported a larger increase in door-to-balloon times compared with high-income countries (19.64 minutes vs 4.52 minutes).

A shift to pharmacologic reperfusion

Over the past 2 decades, there has been a decline in the use of fibrinolytic therapy for STEMI as extensive data demonstrated superior outcomes with PPCI compared with lytic therapy.[21] In the contemporary era, fibrinolytic therapy for STEMI is primarily used only for patients who initially present to a non–PCI-capable hospital with a transfer time to a PCI-capable center of greater than 2 hours. At the beginning of the pandemic, a shift to fibrinolytic therapy was more strongly considered for the management of STEMI even in PPCI-capable hospitals as health care organizations were severely overwhelmed with lack of appropriate resources, anticipated delays in primary PCI, and potential exposure of health care workers.[8,22–24]

In a small case series by Wang and colleagues,[24] 17 STEMI patients who received fibrinolytics were compared with 20 who underwent primary PCI. This study showed comparable in-hospital and 30-day MACE, and mortality rates with no increase in major bleeding risk. By following a modified STEMI care protocol,

where-in fibrinolysis was the preferred treatment of choice for patients with unconfirmed COVID-19 status, intended as an infectious control measure in China at the beginning of the pandemic, Xiang and colleagues[8] reported a dramatic increase in the probability of fibrinolysis as the treatment of choice for STEMI (odds ratio 1.66 [1.50–1.84]), which paralleled a similar decrease in primary PCI rates.

However, this approach has been associated with higher mortality, reinfarction, stroke, and major bleeding.[25,26] Moreover, the benefit of fibrinolytic therapy was negated if there was a considerable delay in presentation, which could result in the formation of a more organized clot that may be resistant to lysis. Although large-scale randomized studies comparing the 2 strategies in the pandemic era are lacking, the rationale for changing the standard of care from PPCI to fibrinolytic therapy has not been clearly established. In addition, the Chinese experience has demonstrated more adverse events with this approach, including death and heart failure, and therefore this shift from mechanical to pharmacologic reperfusion cannot be recommended. Consistent with existing guidelines, a pharmacoinvasive approach can be considered for patients presenting initially to non–PCI-capable hospital when timely transfer to a PCI-capable hospital is not available.[14]

Primary PCI for ST-segment elevation myocardial infarction

Primary percutaneous coronary intervention (PCI), when available and performed by an experienced team in a timely manner, is the preferred reperfusion strategy for treating STEMI to improve survival and reduce rates of recurrent MI and hemorrhagic stroke relative to lytic therapy.[13,21,25] During the pandemic there have been significant reductions in primary PCI rates for STEMI, which paralleled reductions in hospital admissions for STEMI. In The United Kingdom, an 18% reduction in weekly primary PCI rates for STEMI was observed during the first few months of the pandemic compared with the previous year.[18] Similarly, data from the European ISACS-STEMI COVID-19 registry showed a 19% reduction in primary PCI rates between March and April 2020 compared with the same period the previous year.[18] This reduction in procedures was independent of the number of COVID-19 patients.

Despite a significant reduction in overall STEMI admissions in Italy, De Rosa and colleagues[5] noted similar rates of coronary angiography in 2020 compared to 2019 (94.9% vs 94.5%) among those who presented to the hospital with a diagnosis of STEMI, which suggest that the principal barrier to PPCI during the pandemic may be a desire to avoid the health care system during the pandemic, in particular during lockdowns.

Clinical outcomes of ST-segment elevation myocardial infarction patients during the pandemic

Delayed reperfusion in STEMI is associated with larger myocardial scar size, increased risk of heart failure and shock, ventricular arrhythmias, and mortality.[27] There has been an increased risk of mortality and worse outcomes in STEMI patients during the pandemic. STEMI case fatality rate in Italy was 13.7% during the pandemic compared with 4.1% the previous year, a 3-fold increase in mortality.[5] In addition, there was a higher prevalence of major complications (cardiogenic shock, life-threatening arrhythmias, cardiac rupture/ventricular septal defect, and severe functional mitral regurgitation) in these patients during the study period, an increase from 10.4% to 18.8%. In addition, Chew and colleagues[20] demonstrated that there was a higher proportion of patients with post-PCI fibrinolysis in MI thrombolysis in myocardial infarction (TIMI) flow grade less than 3 during the pandemic compared with the prepandemic era indicating suboptimal reperfusion.

In the European ISACS-STEMI COVID-19 registry, the overall in-hospital mortality rate in STEMI patients was significantly higher at 6.8% during the pandemic compared with 4.9% the prior year.[18] This association between the COVID-19 pandemic and higher in-hospital mortality rates persisted even after adjusting for longer total ischemic and door-to-balloon times. There were more late STEMI presentations during the pandemic. Although the true incidence of post-STEMI mechanical complications during the pandemic is currently unknown,[12] Araiza-Garaygordobil and colleagues[28] demonstrated an incidence of 1.98% compared with 0.98% in the prepandemic era in one multinational study, despite similar GRACE risk scores. The increase in short-term complications may lead to prolonged admission to critical care units, which could, in turn, exacerbate a serious shortage in already sparse resources.

Potential causes for worse outcomes in STEMI include prolonged symptom-to-coronary angiography time due to need to test patients for COVID before transport to the CV laboratory, late presentations, reduced rates of primary PCI, and a switch from mechanical to pharmacologic reperfusion. Patients presenting initially to non-PCI hospitals may experience transfer delays or even refusal to transfer due to COVID-19–related health care demands and resource limitations. At the beginning of the pandemic, cardiac catheterization laboratories in some hospitals were suspended to limit exposure until specific hospital-wide protocols were initiated to maintain the safety of personnel and minimize exposure.[14] Also, STEMI protocols were altered during the pandemic to allow for screening and triaging of COVID-19 patients in the emergency department, which could have led to further delays in reperfusion and worse outcomes.[14]

COVID-19 and Non–ST-Segment Elevation Myocardial Infarction

Similar to STEMI, a significant reduction in hospital admissions for NSTEMI has been reported during the pandemic.[3–5] In fact, reductions in hospital admissions and PCI rates for NSTEMI were more pronounced than that seen for STEMI.[6] Compared with a 23% reduction in weekly STEMI admissions, Mafham and colleagues[6] reported a 42% reduction in NSTEMI admissions. Data from Italy showed a 65.4% reduction in hospital admissions for NSTEMI.[5] This was significantly higher compared with a 26.5% reduction in STEMI admissions during the same study period. Solomon and colleagues[4] demonstrated a similar weekly reduction of NSTEMI-related hospital admissions at the beginning of the pandemic in the United States. One possible explanation for this observation is that STEMI patients who present with more severe symptoms tend to seek help more often than patients with NSTEMI.

In a small single-center study, Aldujeli and colleagues[29] reported a significantly longer chest pain-to-door (1885 [880–5732] min vs 606 [388–944] min) and door-to-reperfusion (332 [182–581] min vs 194 [92–329] min) times in NSTEMI patients during the pandemic compared with the prepandemic year. However, clinical outcomes were similar between the groups. Although symptom-to-revascularization time is less frequently studied in patients with NSTEMI/UA, studies have demonstrated worse outcomes in high-risk patients when revascularization is delayed.[30]

A change in revascularization modalities has also occurred during the pandemic. Mafham and colleagues[6] observed that NSTEMI patients were more likely to undergo PCI rather than coronary artery bypass graft surgery (CABG) surgery (up to 80% reduction in CABG surgery), which was in line with the recommendations from the British Cardiovascular Intervention Society to minimize utilization of intensive care unit beds. Moreover, there was also a paucity of mechanical ventilators because of the diversion of resources to critically ill COVID-19 patients. Interestingly, these patients received PCI more often on the day of admission resulting in a shorter length of hospital stays, to minimize exposure and make beds available for sicker COVID-19 patients. Despite this shift away from CABG surgery, there was a 37% reduction in weekly PCI rates for NSTEMI during the pandemic compared with the year prior.

In addition to reduced hospitalizations and prolonged symptom-to-revascularization times, the rate of major complications (cardiogenic shock, life-threatening arrhythmias, cardiac rupture/ventricular septal defect, and severe functional mitral regurgitation) was reported to have increased from 5.1% to 10.7% in NSTEMI in one study.[5]

Acute Myocardial Infarction Care in COVID-19 Patients

Myocardial injury, defined as an elevation in troponin levels above the 99th percentile, is common in hospitalized patients with COVID-19 infection with an incidence ranging between 8% and 36% (see Laura De Michieli and colleagues' article, "Use and Prognostic Implications of Cardiac Troponin in COVID-19," in this issue).[31,32] The incidence of myocardial injury parallels the severity of COVID-19 infection with a 13-fold increase in risk among patients in intensive care units.[31] Troponin elevation in COVID-19 is independently associated with increased risk of mortality, especially for those with underlying history of cardiovascular disease.[33,34] Differential diagnoses for elevated troponin in COVID-19 include acute MI, microvascular thrombosis, acute heart failure, myocarditis, stress-induced cardiomyopathy, supply-demand mismatch, disseminated intravascular coagulation, cytokine storm, and lastly acute pulmonary embolism.[35]

COVID-19 may increase the risk of acute MI with a reported incidence between 1.1% and 8.9%.[36,37] The risk is higher in the first 2 weeks after infection with Modin and colleagues[38] showing an approximately 5-fold increased risk. A large population-based study of all COVID-19 patients in Sweden reported that the risk of acute MI in these patients is significantly higher in the first 1 week after exposure and subsequently decreases by weeks 2 and 3.[39] The pathophysiology of acute MI in COVID-19 includes (1) increased risk of plaque rupture and thrombosis (type 1 AMI) or (2) myocardial oxygen imbalance due to supply-demand mismatch (type 2 AMI). This is attributed to the intense systemic inflammatory response and a relative prothrombotic state caused by the SARS-CoV-2 virus.[40]

The diagnosis of acute MI become more challenging for clinicians around the world during these unprecedented times. In COVID-19 patients, it is crucial to differentiate ACS and myocardial injury as treatment varies significantly. Although the same criteria can be used to diagnose STEMI in COVID-19 patients compared with the general population, the diagnosis of NSTEMI can be particularly challenging as troponin elevation is commonly seen in these patients. COVID-19 patients presenting with acute MI may have complex coronary anatomy with higher thrombus burden, lesion haziness, ulcerative lesions, and prevalence of multivessel CAD.[41] The prothrombotic state associated with COVID-19 infection could possibly play a role in a higher thrombus burden in acute MI patients.

Early in the pandemic, De Rosa and colleagues[5] reported that among all STEMI patients, 10.7% were COVID+ with a case fatality rate of 28.6% compared with 11% in COVID patients. Similarly, in-hospital mortality from STEMI in COVID-19 patients was 29% in the European ISACS-STEMI COVID-19 registry.[18] The North American COVID-19 Myocardial Infarction (NACMI) registry, a prospective, multicenter, observational registry of hospitalized STEMI patients with confirmed COVID-19 infection comprehensively evaluated patient characteristics in this high-risk population.[42] This important registry has shown that 1 in 5 COVID-19 patients with STEMI did not undergo invasive coronary angiogram and among those who did about 1 in 4 had normal coronary arteries. In addition, the study demonstrated that despite having a high-risk presentation with more cardiogenic shock, COVID-19 patients were less likely to undergo PCI (71% vs 100%), had significantly longer door-to-balloon times (79 min vs 66 min), and significantly higher in-hospital mortality (33% vs 4%) compared with age- and sex-matched historical controls. Despite this, primary PCI remained the preferred revascularization strategy in these patients with a 48% mortality among those who did not undergo coronary angiogram compared with 28% among those who did. This highlights the feasibility of primary PCI in COVID-19 patients, which remains the recommended modality of revascularization in STEMI.[13]

The European Association for Cardiovascular Imaging (EACVI) and the American Association of Cardiology (ACC) have highlighted recommendations to help guide clinicians in making appropriate decisions with regard to caring for patients suspected or diagnosed to have COVID-related acute myocardial injury.[14,43] Acute MI care in COVID-19 patients is discussed in detail in Thomas A. Kite and colleagues' article, "The Direct and Indirect

Effects of COVID-19 on Acute Coronary Syndromes," in this issue.

Initiatives to Improve Acute Myocardial Infarction Care and Future Directions

It is clear that the COVID-19 pandemic continues to have a negative impact on acute MI care. Conceptually, the COVID-19 pandemic has had direct (increased arterial and venous thrombogenicity, troponin elevation, microthrombi, respiratory failure, in-hospital presentation) and indirect effects (lockdowns, cancellation of services, restrictive visitation policies, delayed presentations) on acute MI care, which collectively have resulted in increased morbidity and mortality.[44,45]

A thorough understanding of the barriers to seeking and providing cardiovascular care in acute MI during this pandemic is crucial to improving outcomes. Primary PCI continues to be the preferred treatment of choice in STEMI patients and studies have demonstrated worse outcomes in those who did not receive primary PCI during the pandemic.[22] COVID-19 may remain in the community for the foreseeable future, especially in light of mutations creating newer variants of the SARS-CoV-2 virus with a higher infectivity rate and complications. As vaccines have become available, clinical presentations of vaccinated COVID-19 patients may differ from the unvaccinated. Campaigns such as SCAI's Seconds Still Count have reversed early declines in STEMI presentations and should be expanded.[9] The use of social and other media to bring awareness about the importance of timely reperfusion should be emphasized. It is clear that restrictive lockdowns are detrimental for health care delivery and more circumspect approaches are needed.[44] For effective results, such campaigns should be able to cross cultural, socioeconomic, and psychosocial barriers. Strategies for emergency network reorganization, including rapid screening of acute MI patients and appropriate allocation of resources for critically ill non-COVID patients, are also needed. System-wide standardized protocols need to be implemented by health care organizations to ensure rapid, and safe access to health care in a timely manner for improved outcomes in acute MI while ensuring the safety of the health care personnel.

Interruptions in critical health care services have been reported during prior epidemics/pandemics. The American Heart Association issued temporary emergency guidance on STEMI care that included improving awareness among the general public about the symptoms and signs of "heart attack," screening patients for COVID symptoms, identifying STEMI mimics before catheterization laboratory activation, and minimizing delays to primary PCI for clear STEMI while testing for COVID-19.[46] PCI was recommended as the preferred primary reperfusion strategy in these patients irrespective of their COVID status. The Society for Cardiovascular Angiography and Interventions (SCAI), the American College of Cardiology (ACC), and the American College of Emergency Physicians (ACEP) advocate that those patients needing emergency cardiac catheterization should be treated as possible COVID-19 and treated accordingly pending testing.[14] Cardiovascular societies and health care organizations need to continue to work together to formulate pragmatic guidelines and protocols with the goal of delivering the best possible care for acute MI patients while maintaining the safety of hospital personnel in these troubled times.

SUMMARY

The COVID-19 pandemic has resulted in restricted access to clinical services and worse clinical outcomes for patients with acute MI. The mechanisms are multifactorial and include avoidance of medical care during lockdowns, late presentations, reorganization of treatment pathways—including deviations from standard of care protocols during COVID surges—, and a shift from mechanical to pharmacologic reperfusion. Many of these trends have the potential to undo 3 decades of progress in STEMI care and therefore must be reversed in a timely manner. Educational campaigns such as SCAI's Seconds Still Count have reversed early declines in STEMI presentations and should be replicated and expanded.

CLINICS CARE POINTS

- Timely primary percutaneous coronary intervention remains the dominant revascularization modality for STEMI patients during the pandemic.

DISCLOSURE

Dr S. Garcia is a consultant for Medtronic, Edwards Lifesciences, BSCI, and Abbott Vascular; has received institutional research grants from Edwards Lifesciences, Abbott Vascular, Gore, and BSCI; and is a proctor for Edwards Lifesciences. The other authors have nothing to disclose.

REFERENCES

1. Benjamin EJ, Muntner P, Alonso A, et al. Heart disease and stroke statistics-2019 update: a report from the american heart association. Circulation 2019;139(10):e56–528.

2. Garcia S, Albaghdadi MS, Meraj PM, et al. Reduction in ST-segment elevation cardiac catheterization laboratory activations in the United States during COVID-19 pandemic. J Am Coll Cardiol 2020; 75(22):2871–2.

3. De Filippo O, D'Ascenzo F, Angelini F, et al. Reduced rate of hospital admissions for ACS during Covid-19 outbreak in northern Italy. N Engl J Med 2020;383(1):88–9.

4. Solomon MD, McNulty EJ, Rana JS, et al. The Covid-19 pandemic and the incidence of acute myocardial infarction. N Engl J Med 2020;383(7):691–3.

5. De Rosa S, Spaccarotella C, Basso C, et al. Reduction of hospitalizations for myocardial infarction in Italy in the COVID-19 era. Eur Heart J 2020;41(22): 2083–8.

6. Mafham MM, Spata E, Goldacre R, et al. COVID-19 pandemic and admission rates for and management of acute coronary syndromes in England. Lancet 2020;396(10248):381–9.

7. Mohammad MA, Koul S, Olivecrona GK, et al. Incidence and outcome of myocardial infarction treated with percutaneous coronary intervention during COVID-19 pandemic. Heart 2020;106(23):1812–8.

8. Xiang D, Xiang X, Zhang W, et al. Management and outcomes of patients with STEMI during the COVID-19 pandemic in China. J Am Coll Cardiol 2020; 76(11):1318–24.

9. Garcia S, Stanberry L, Schmidt C, et al. Impact of COVID-19 pandemic on STEMI care: an expanded analysis from the United States. Catheter Cardiovasc Interv 2021;98(2):217–22.

10. Abdelaziz HK, Abdelrahman A, Nabi A, et al. Impact of COVID-19 pandemic on patients with ST-segment elevation myocardial infarction: insights from a British cardiac center. Am Heart J 2020;226:45–8.

11. Lai PH, Lancet EA, Weiden MD, et al. Characteristics associated with out-of-hospital cardiac arrests and resuscitations during the novel coronavirus disease 2019 pandemic in New York city. JAMA Cardiol 2020;5(10):1154–63.

12. Riley RF, Kereiakes DJ, Mahmud E, et al. Back to the future" for STEMI?: the COVID-19 experience. JACC Case Rep 2020;2(10):1651–3.

13. Nallamothu BK, Normand SL, Wang Y, et al. Relation between door-to-balloon times and mortality after primary percutaneous coronary intervention over time: a retrospective study. Lancet 2015;385(9973): 1114–22.

14. Mahmud E, Dauerman HL, FGP Welt, et al. Management of acute myocardial infarction during the COVID-19 pandemic: a position statement from the society for cardiovascular angiography and interventions (SCAI), the american college of cardiology (ACC), and the american college of emergency physicians (ACEP). J Am Coll Cardiol 2020;76(11): 1375–84.

15. De Luca G, van 't Hof AW, de Boer MJ, et al. Time-to-treatment significantly affects the extent of ST-segment resolution and myocardial blush in patients with acute myocardial infarction treated by primary angioplasty. Eur Heart J 2004;25(12):1009–13.

16. De Luca G, Suryapranata H, Ottervanger JP, et al. Time delay to treatment and mortality in primary angioplasty for acute myocardial infarction: every minute of delay counts. Circulation 2004;109(10): 1223–5.

17. Terkelsen CJ, Sørensen JT, Maeng M, et al. System delay and mortality among patients with STEMI treated with primary percutaneous coronary intervention. JAMA 2010;304(7):763–71.

18. De Luca G, Verdoia M, Cercek M, et al. Impact of COVID-19 pandemic on mechanical reperfusion for patients with STEMI. J Am Coll Cardiol 2020; 76(20):2321–30.

19. Lechner I, Reindl M, Tiller C, et al. Impact of COVID-19 pandemic restrictions on ST-elevation myocardial infarction: a cardiac magnetic resonance imaging study. European Heart Journal 2021;43:1141–53.

20. Chew NWS, Ow ZGW, Teo VXY, et al. The global effect of the COVID-19 pandemic on STEMI care: a systematic review and meta-analysis. Can J Cardiol 2021;37(9):1450–9.

21. Keeley EC, Boura JA, Grines CL. Primary angioplasty versus intravenous thrombolytic therapy for acute myocardial infarction: a quantitative review of 23 randomised trials. Lancet 2003;361(9351): 13–20.

22. Jing ZC, Zhu HD, Yan XW, et al. Recommendations from the peking union medical college hospital for the management of acute myocardial infarction during the COVID-19 outbreak. Eur Heart J 2020; 41(19):1791–4.

23. Zhang L, Fan Y, Lu Z. Experiences and lesson strategies for cardiology from the COVID-19 outbreak in Wuhan, China, by 'on the scene' cardiologists. Eur Heart J 2020;41(19):1788–90.

24. Wang N, Zhang M, Su H, et al. Fibrinolysis is a reasonable alternative for STEMI care during the COVID-19 pandemic. J Int Med Res 2020;48(10). 300060520966151.

25. Stenestrand U, Lindback J, Wallentin L, et al. Long-term outcome of primary percutaneous coronary intervention vs prehospital and in-hospital thrombolysis for patients with ST-elevation myocardial infarction. JAMA 2006;296(14):1749–56.

26. Huynh T, Perron S, O'Loughlin J, et al. Comparison of primary percutaneous coronary intervention and

fibrinolytic therapy in ST-segment-elevation myocardial infarction: bayesian hierarchical meta-analyses of randomized controlled trials and observational studies. Circulation 2009;119(24):3101–9.

27. St John Sutton M, Lee D, Rouleau JL, et al. Left ventricular remodeling and ventricular arrhythmias after myocardial infarction. Circulation 2003;107(20):2577–82.

28. Araiza-Garaygordobil D, Montalto C, Martinez-Amezcua P, et al. Impact of the COVID-19 pandemic on hospitalizations for acute coronary syndromes: a multinational study. QJM 2021;114(9):642–7.

29. Aldujeli A, Hamadeh A, Briedis K, et al. Delays in Presentation in patients with acute myocardial infarction during the COVID-19 pandemic. Cardiol Res 2020;11(6):386–91.

30. Case BC, Yerasi C, Wang Y, et al. Admissions rate and timing of revascularization in the United States in patients with Non-ST-elevation myocardial infarction. Am J Cardiol 2020;134:24–31.

31. Li B, Yang J, Zhao F, et al. Prevalence and impact of cardiovascular metabolic diseases on COVID-19 in China. Clin Res Cardiol 2020;109(5):531–8.

32. Lala A, Johnson KW, Januzzi JL, et al. Prevalence and impact of myocardial injury in patients hospitalized with COVID-19 infection. J Am Coll Cardiol 2020;76(5):533–46.

33. Zheng YY, Ma YT, Zhang JY, et al. COVID-19 and the cardiovascular system. Nat Rev Cardiol 2020;17(5):259–60.

34. Guo T, Fan Y, Chen M, et al. Cardiovascular implications of fatal outcomes of patients with Coronavirus disease 2019 (COVID-19). JAMA Cardiol 2020;5(7):811–8.

35. Madjid M, Safavi-Naeini P, Solomon SD, et al. Potential Effects of coronaviruses on the cardiovascular system: a review. JAMA Cardiol 2020;5(7):831–40.

36. Lodigiani C, Iapichino G, Carenzo L, et al. Venous and arterial thromboembolic complications in COVID-19 patients admitted to an academic hospital in Milan, Italy. Thromb Res 2020;191:9–14.

37. Bilaloglu S, Aphinyanaphongs Y, Jones S, et al. Thrombosis in hospitalized patients with COVID-19 in a New York City health system. JAMA 2020;324(8):799–801.

38. Modin D, Claggett B, Sindet-Pedersen C, et al. Acute COVID-19 and the incidence of ischemic stroke and acute myocardial infarction. Circulation 2020;142(21):2080–2.

39. Katsoularis I, Fonseca-Rodriguez O, Farrington P, et al. Risk of acute myocardial infarction and ischaemic stroke following COVID-19 in Sweden: a self-controlled case series and matched cohort study. Lancet 2021;398(10300):599–607.

40. Becker RC. COVID-19 update: covid-19-associated coagulopathy. J Thromb Thrombolysis 2020;50(1):54–67.

41. Abizaid A, Campos CM, Guimaraes PO, et al. Patients with COVID-19 who experience a myocardial infarction have complex coronary morphology and high in-hospital mortality: primary results of a nationwide angiographic study. Catheter Cardiovasc Interv 2021;98(3):E370–8.

42. Garcia S, Dehghani P, Grines C, et al. Initial findings from the North American COVID-19 myocardial infarction registry. J Am Coll Cardiol 2021;77(16):1994–2003.

43. Skulstad H, Cosyns B, Popescu BA, et al. COVID-19 pandemic and cardiac imaging: EACVI recommendations on precautions, indications, prioritization, and protection for patients and healthcare personnel. Eur Heart J Cardiovasc Imaging 2020;21(6):592–8.

44. Henry TD, Kereiakes DJ. The direct and indirect effects of the COVID-19 pandemic on cardiovascular disease throughout the world. Eur Heart J 2021;ehab782.

45. American heart association's mission L, get with the guidelines coronary artery disease advisory work G, the council on clinical cardiology's committees on acute cardiac C, general C, interventional cardiovascular C. Temporary emergency guidance to STEMI systems of care during the COVID-19 pandemic: AHA's mission: lifeline. Circulation 2020;142(3):199–202.

46. Sofi F, Dinu M, Reboldi G, et al. Worldwide differences of hospitalization for ST-segment elevation myocardial infarction during COVID-19: a systematic review and meta-analysis. Int J Cardiol 2022;347:89–96.

Impact of Coronavirus Disease 2019 Pandemic on Cardiac Arrest and Emergency Care

Murtaza Bharmal, MD[a], Kyle DiGrande, MD[a], Akash Patel, MD[a], David M. Shavelle, MD[b], Nichole Bosson, MD, MPH, NRP, FAEMS[c,d,e],*

KEYWORDS

- Cardiac arrest • Emergency care • Out-of-hospital cardiac arrest • In-hospital cardiac arrest
- COVID-19 pandemic

KEY POINTS

- The COVID-19 pandemic has increased the incidence of both out-of-hospital and in-hospital cardiac arrest.
- The increase in the incidence of cardiac arrest seems to be multifactorial and related to the severity of COVID-19 in the community, reduced access to health care, and patient delays in seeking care.
- During the COVID-19 pandemic, patient survival and neurologic outcome after both out-of-hospital and in-hospital cardiac arrest were reduced.
- The worse outcome may be related to a combination of factors including reduction in bystander cardiopulmonary resuscitation rates, delays in emergency medical system response times and transport, higher incidence of nonshockable rhythms, and reduced access to emergency and in-hospital care because of COVID-19-related hospitalizations.
- A better understanding of the mechanisms by which COVID-19 has disrupted the chain of survival can direct further effort to mitigate the negative impacts on cardiac arrest and patient outcome. Understanding how the system response to a pandemic can be modified to increase lives saved is essential.

INTRODUCTION

Cardiac arrest continues to be a major public health concern. In the United States, the incidence of out-of-hospital cardiac arrest (OHCA) and in-hospital cardiac arrest (IHCA) are approximately 350,000 and 200,000 per year, respectively.[1,2] Despite significant advances in other areas of cardiovascular medicine, survival from cardiac arrest remains low.[3] Effective treatment of cardiac arrest includes bystander cardiopulmonary resuscitation (CPR), early activation of emergency medical services (EMS), early defibrillation, advanced cardiovascular life support, and postresuscitation care that includes targeted temperature management and emergency coronary angiography with percutaneous coronary intervention in some cases.

This article originally appeared in Cardiology Clinics, Volume 40, Issue 3, August 2022.
[a] Department of Cardiology, University of California Irvine Medical Center, 510 E Peltason Drive, Irvine, CA 92697, USA; [b] MemorialCare Heart and Vascular Institute, Long Beach Medical Center, 2801 Atlantic Avenue, Long Beach, CA 90807, USA; [c] Los Angeles County Emergency Medical Services Agency, 10100 Pioneer Boulevard Ste 200, Santa Fe Springs, CA 90670, USA; [d] Department of Emergency Medicine, Harbor-UCLA Medical Center, 1000 W Carson Street, Torrance, CA, 90509, USA; [e] David Geffen School of Medicine at UCLA, 10833 Le Conte Avenue, Los Angeles, CA 90095, USA
* Corresponding author. Los Angeles County EMS Agency, Los Angeles County Emergency Medical Services, 10100 Pioneer Boulevard Ste 200, Santa Fe Springs, CA 90670.
E-mail address: Nbosson@dhs.lacounty.gov

Heart Failure Clin 19 (2023) 231–240
https://doi.org/10.1016/j.hfc.2022.08.009

Since the emergence of COVID-19 and the global pandemic declared by the World Health Organization on March 11, 2020, there have been more than 230 million confirmed cases around the world with more than 4.8 million deaths.[4] The COVID-19 pandemic has affected the incidence, presentation, care, and outcome of time-sensitive medical conditions including cardiac arrest.[5] Beyond the direct mortality related to the respiratory infection, health care systems have been overwhelmed by COVID-19-related hospitalizations, disruptions to the work force because of infected health care personnel, and logistical challenges related to implementation of strategies to minimize disease transmission. A reduction in elective cardiovascular procedures, shortened length of hospital stay, and longer delays between symptom onset and hospital treatment have also been observed during the COVID-19 pandemic.[6] In this article, the effects of the COVID-19 pandemic on cardiac arrest are presented, considering data from recent clinical studies, with a focus on the contributing factors and implications for improving outcome.

OUT-OF-HOSPITAL CARDIAC ARREST
Incidence

During the COVID-19 pandemic, the incidence of OHCA significantly increased with multiple geographic regions throughout the world reporting similar trends.[7–12] In the United States, various regions noted an increase in OHCA. Rollman and colleagues[7] reported a 21% increase in the incidence of OHCA in Los Angeles County, CA, USA, a diverse population of approximately 10.1 million persons. Matthew and colleagues[9] found a 62% increase in Detroit, MI, USA, using data from the Cardiac Arrest Registry to Enhance Survival (CARES). Lai and colleagues[12] reported an approximately 3-fold higher incidence of OHCA in New York City, NY, USA, a particularly hard-hit area early in the pandemic, which is also among the largest EMS systems in the United States serving a population of approximately 8.4 million (**Fig. 1**). Similarly, in Europe, Baldi and colleagues[10] analyzed data from the Lombardi Cardiac Arrest Registry that included 4 providences in Italy and found a 58% increase in OHCA. Marion and colleagues[8] found a 2-fold increase in OHCA in Paris, France, and the surrounding suburbs. In a meta-analysis of 10 studies with more than 35,000 OHCA events in various geographic regions, Lim and colleagues[13] found a 120% increase in OHCA.

In contrast to the aforementioned studies, several studies found no increase in OHCA.[11,14–16]

Huber and colleagues[11] found no significant increase in OHCA within a community in Germany with a low prevalence of COVID-19 infection. Elmer and colleagues[15] also reported no significant increase in OHCA in Pennsylvania, USA, where the prevalence of COVID-19 was low. Chan and colleagues[17] observed communities with different COVID-19 mortality rates and found the incidence of OHCA was higher largely in communities with high COVID-19 mortality. Although these studies in aggregate suggest that the incidence of OHCA is related to the prevalence of COVID-19 infection within the community, it does not follow that patients experiencing OHCA were predominately COVID-19 positive.[18]

Patient and Arrest Characteristics

During the COVID-19 pandemic, there were also notable changes in baseline patient characteristics among those experiencing OHCA. Lai and colleagues[12] found that patients were older, less likely to be white, and more likely to have comorbid conditions, including diabetes mellitus and hypertension, compared with a prepandemic control group. Nonshockable rhythms (asystole and pulseless electrical activity) were also more common. Sultanian and colleagues[19] further evaluated the association between COVID-19 and the initial arrest rhythm; patients with confirmed COVID-19 were less likely to have a shockable rhythm compared with patients who were known to be COVID-19 negative. While Marijon and colleagues[8] did not note significant differences in baseline characteristics, the investigators observed higher rates of OHCA occurring at home, less frequent bystander CPR, and less frequent shockable rhythms. Two systematic reviews, one by Scquizzato and colleagues[20] that included 6 studies and another by Lim and colleagues with many of the same and totaling 10 studies found lower rates of shockable rhythm, lower rates of witnessed arrests, and lower rates of bystander CPR.[21]

Out-of-Hospital Arrest Management

OHCA is a time-critical emergency, with reduced chance of survival for every minute of delay. Multiple studies documented increased EMS response and transport times during the COVID-19 pandemic.[6,8,18,20,22,23] Use of personal protective equipment (PPE) to ensure health care provider safety and reduce transmission of COVID-19 during on-scene resuscitation likely contributed to delays in treatment and transport.[24] Furthermore, workforce reduction due to illness and overwhelmed health care systems leading to longer

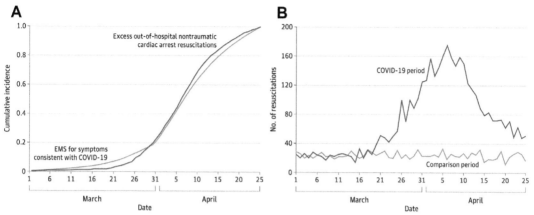

Fig. 1. New York City out-of-hospital nontraumatic cardiac arrest resuscitations, March 1 through April 25, 2020. (*A*) Temporal association between the cumulative percentage of EMS calls for fever, cough, dyspnea, and virallike symptoms consistent with coronavirus disease 2019 (COVID-19) and the number of excess out-of-hospital non-traumatic cardiac arrest resuscitations occurring in New York City in 2020. Excess cases were defined as the daily difference between the number of 2020 and 2019 cases; days with a negative difference were recoded as 0 for graphic presentation. (*B*) The number of daily out-of-hospital nontraumatic cardiac arrest resuscitations. (*From* Lai, P.H., et al., Characteristics Associated With Out-of-Hospital Cardiac Arrests and Resuscitations During the Novel Coronavirus Disease 2019 Pandemic in New York City. JAMA Cardiol, 2020. 5(10): p. 1154-1163.)

patient offload times at the hospital resulted in less available resources to respond to time-sensitive emergencies. Changes in resuscitation protocols during the COVID-19 pandemic by various EMS systems in response to resource limitations as well as uncertainties early in the pandemic may have affected prehospital management, response, and transport times.[22,25] Early recommendations, when PPE was scarce, included limiting personnel during the resuscitation, which could have had implications for outcome, and considering the appropriateness of initiation resuscitation.[26] Congruent with the observation of less frequent shockable rhythms, rates of defibrillation were significantly lower during the COVID-19 pandemic.[7] Studies also documented a reduction in attempted resuscitation measures[8]; this was again likely driven by the increase in unfavorable prognostic factors, although a fear of disease transmission by first responders, lack of EMS and hospital resources, and a perception of poor prognosis for COVID-positive patients experiencing OHCA may have contributed.

Outcome

Studies reporting outcome events during the COVID-19 pandemic were consistent and documented lower rates of return of spontaneous circulation (ROSC), less frequent survival to hospital admission, lower survival to hospital discharge, and worse neurologic outcome.[8,9,12,13,20] The prevalence of COVID-19 infection within the

community also seems to be associated with worse outcome for those experiencing OHCA.[17] Chan and colleagues[17] used data from CARES throughout the United States to evaluate the association between OHCA outcomes and the COVID-19 disease burden within geographic areas; whereas ROSC was lower regardless of COVID-19 burden, survival to hospital discharge was primarily lower in communities with moderate to very high COVID-19 mortality rates.

IN-HOSPITAL CARDIAC ARREST
Incidence

Although data are limited, the incidence of IHCA in the United States before the COVID-19 pandemic was estimated at 10 per 1000 admissions.[27] This incidence varies by county and region with reports from the United Kingdom, for example, estimating an incidence of 1.6 per 1000 admissions making comparisons with current pandemic rates challenging.[28] Most recent literature has focused on IHCA occurring among COVID-19-positive patients. The incidence of IHCA seems to have increased during the COVID-19 pandemic, driven by high mortality among patients with COVID-19 and a decrease in hospitalizations for other conditions.[29–33] At the onset of the pandemic, Shao and colleagues[29] reported that 20% experienced IHCA in a consecutive series of patients from Wuhan, China, who required hospitalization for COVID-19 pneumonia. Subsequently, reports from New York in the United States of hospitalized patients with COVID-19 found IHCA rates of 3% to 7%.[30,31] However, among critically ill patients with COVID-19 in the intensive care unit (ICU), IHCA was more frequent. In a multicenter study from the United States of more than 5000 critically ill patients with COVID-19, 14% suffered IHCA.[32]

The few reports evaluating IHCA rates in non-COVID patients are mixed.[33] In a separate analysis from the aforementioned study, Roedl and colleagues[33] reported a decline in overall hospital admission in Germany during the peak of the pandemic, with an increase in IHCA among all hospitalized patients from the prepandemic era of 4.6% to 6.6% during the pandemic. However, both COVID-positive and COVID-negative patients were included in this study. In a study of only COVID-negative patients in Hong Kong, Tong and colleagues[34] found a decline in IHCA from 1.6 to 1.4 per 1000 admissions before and during the pandemic.

Patient and Arrest Characteristics

Baseline characteristics for patients with IHCA were different during the COVID-19 pandemic compared with the prepandemic era. Studies within the United States found an increased prevalence of IHCA among minorities (black and Hispanic patients) during the COVID-19 pandemic compared with earlier control periods.[30] In addition, studies from multiple geographic regions consistently found a higher prevalence of cardiovascular disease and cardiovascular risk factors in patients with IHCA during the COVID-19 pandemic compared with control periods.[29,31–33] In an evaluation before the pandemic, Andersen and colleagues[28] reported that the underlying cause of arrest was primary cardiac (50%–60%) followed by respiratory. In contrast, the most common cause for arrest in most studies during the pandemic was respiratory and most patients were intubated before the arrest.[29,31,35] Most studies found low rates of a shockable rhythm during the COVID-19 pandemic, ranging from 3% to 18%, similar to prepandemic data.[19,29–32,36] Rates of CPR within the aforementioned studies varied from 50% to 90%.[29,32] In general, time to treatment and resuscitation times were similar during the COVID-19 period compared with prior years.[31,33] When comparing the pandemic period to prepandemic, IHCA more commonly occurred in a general medical ward (as opposed to ICU) in some studies,[29,31] although other studies found higher rates of ICU IHCA during the pandemic.[33] Although location of the arrest has implications for recognition and response time, it may also reflect hospital overcrowding and conversion of non-ICU beds to a semi-ICU setting in some hospital systems and, therefore, would vary by region.

In-Hospital Cardiac Arrest Management

Early in the pandemic, there were little data to inform management. Prone positioning of patients with severe COVID-19, as well as the logistics of maintaining isolation precautions, added further challenges to achieving rapid response and high-quality resuscitation. Several novel treatment approaches were suggested for IHCA during the COVID-19 pandemic, including increased use of mechanical CPR devices, performance of prone CPR, and application of extracorporeal membrane oxygenation (ECMO).[37–39] Each of these presents its own challenges and are not feasible in all health care settings. There are limited data on outcome from prone CPR; however, it has the advantage to reduce delays to initiation of compressions as well as minimizing the complications that could occur from attempting repositioning in the prone patient.[38] ECMO rapidly became a limited resource given the high burden of COVID-19 in many communities and the need for specialty centers with expertise to manage these complicated patients. As such, use of ECMO has been limited to patients with COVID-19 not in cardiac arrest or patients with other causes of IHCA with an overall better prognosis and/or a clear, treatable underlying condition.[37,40]

Outcome

IHCA has a high mortality.[28] Similar to the findings for OHCA, studies reporting outcome events for IHCA during the COVID-19 pandemic were consistent and documented lower rates of ROSC, lower survival to hospital discharge, and worse neurologic outcome.[29,31,32] Survival to hospital discharge ranged from 0% to 14%.[31,32,36] During the peak of the COVID-19 pandemic in Wuhan, China, Shao and colleagues[29] reported 30-day survival of only 2.9%. Hayek and colleagues[32] reported data from a large multicenter registry from the United States and found that survival to hospital discharge was associated with patient age; for those younger than 45 years, survival was 21% compared with only 3% for those older than 80 years. A meta-analysis by Ippolito and colleagues[41] that included 7 studies, with all patients receiving attempted resuscitation, found an in-hospital survival rate of approximately 4%. These low survival rates have led some to question the benefits of performing CPR on patients with COVID-19.[33,42] However, the ability to predict outcome for patients with IHCA is challenging. The GO-FAR Score (Good Outcome Following

Attempted Resuscitation) is a validated scoring system that uses prearrest variables to predict the probability of survival to hospital discharge following IHCA.[43] In the aforementioned study by Aldabagh and colleagues[30] actual survival was compared with the GO-FAR score in 450 patients with IHCA. Unfortunately, COVID-19-positive patients had lower observed survival than predicted by the GO-FAR Score. However, lower survival rates are not entirely consistent across studies; Roedl and colleagues[33] found higher survival in COVID-positive versus COVID-negative patients with IHCA due to respiratory failure, albeit among a small cohort of 43 patients.

The low survival rates for IHCA seems to be multifactorial, related to the presence of the underlying illness at the time of arrest (mechanical ventilation, kidney replacement therapy, or vasopressor support), a high percentage of non-shockable rhythms, lack of therapies to treat the underlying disease process, and potential delays in response time because of isolation procedures, the need to use PPE, and restricted access to COVID-19 units. Improving outcomes of IHCA in patients with COVID-19 will be challenging, because many of the factors associated with poor outcome may not be modifiable. Further investigation into the risks and benefits of performing prolonged CPR in this subset of patients is needed, especially related to the concern for increased aerosolization of viral particles that places health care personnel at increased risk of contracting the infection.

MECHANISM FOR INCREASED CARDIAC ARREST

Multiple different mechanisms have been proposed to explain how the COVID-19 pandemic may have led to the increased incidence and worse outcomes from cardiac arrest. A dichotomy that includes both the direct and indirect effects of COVID-19 is a useful framework to understand this complex interaction[18] (**Table 1**).

Direct Effects of COVID-19

COVID-19 can lead to the occurrence of cardiac arrest throughout multiple pathways. First, the respiratory illness itself with progressive hypoxia from ongoing pneumonia and acute respiratory distress syndrome can trigger cardiac arrest. In addition, particularly in the advanced stages of disease, COVID-19 progresses to a systemic endothelial inflammatory illness with an exaggerated immune response and cytokine storm.[44,45] In patients with preexisting cardiac conditions, this high inflammatory burden may induce vascular

Table 1 Direct and indirect effects of coronavirus disease 2019 on cardiac arrest	
Direct Effects	**Indirect Effects**
• Respiratory illness leading to hypoxia • Endothelial inflammatory illness • Exaggerated immune response • Cytokine storm • Vascular thrombosis • Myocarditis • Arrhythmias • Prothrombotic state triggering pulmonary embolism and acute coronary syndrome • Drug treatment causing risk for arrhythmias	• Stringent lockdown measures • Stay-at-home order • Health care reorganization • Reduction in preventive and emergent diagnostic testing and procedures • Overwhelmed EMS and hospital systems • Use of personal protective equipment • Reduction in hospital work force • Delay in patient care • At-risk patients alone more often

Abbreviation: EMS, emergency medical system.

thrombosis, myocarditis, and cardiac arrhythmias.[46] Even in patients without predisposing conditions, a significant prothrombotic state has been associated with COVID-19 infections with an increased incidence in thromboembolic events including pulmonary embolism and acute coronary syndrome, possibly increasing the risk of cardiac arrest, particularly in the setting of concomitant inflammation.[47,48] Various drug treatments including hydroxychloroquine and azithromycin may further increase the risk of cardiac arrest, particularly in patients with preexisting cardiac conditions.[49]

Indirect Effects of COVID-19

Despite the potential direct effects of COVID-19 on cardiac arrest, the proportion of patients with OHCA with active and/or confirmed COVID-19 infection seems to be relatively low. For example, confirmed and suspected cases of COVID-19 in a French population accounted for only 30% of the observed increase in the incidence of OHCA.[8] Data from the Victorian Ambulance Cardiac Arrest Registry cross-referenced with the Victorian Department of Health and Human Services COVID registry demonstrated less public arrest, less public access defibrillation, lower rates of resuscitation by EMS, longer time to key intervention (defibrillation, epinephrine), and a 50% reduction in survival despite none of the patients in the registry testing positive for COVID-19.[50] These data suggest that the indirect effects may play an equal or even more important role in the increased incidence in and worse outcome from cardiac arrest observed during the COVID-19 pandemic. The potential indirect effects include stringent lockdowns and stay-at-home messaging, health care reorganization, reductions in preventive and emergency procedures, and overwhelmed EMS and hospital systems.

Lockdowns and movement restrictions, along with fear of seeking medical care due to potential exposure to COVID-19, made patients reluctant to seek emergency services, resulting in delayed care and worse outcome. Social restrictions and self-isolation during the pandemic likely caused at-risk patients to be alone more often, thus reducing the occurrence of witnessed arrests and reducing the possibility of bystander CPR[18,51]; this is consistent with a prior study that documented that those living alone were more likely to present with severe complaints and have an increased risk for early mortality.[52] Friedman and Akrenoted a striking increase in overdose-related deaths early in the pandemic, likely due to social isolation leading to both an increased use of substances due to stressors and use of substances while alone.[53]

The COVID-19 pandemic shifted the focus of health care to treatment of those afflicted with the acute respiratory infection while attempting to minimize the spread; this required changes to non-COVID medical care. Health care systems reorganized to accommodate the massive surge of patients with a highly infectious disease. Elective procedures including echocardiograms, cardiovascular stress tests, and coronary angiography were canceled to reallocate resources to COVID-19 treatment, as well as to avoid unnecessary exposure to stable and at-risk patients. During the pandemic, hospitalization rates for congestive heart failure, acute myocardial infarction, and arrhythmias were all lower than those during pre-COVID control periods.[54] Without timely hospitalization and/or prompt medical care, these cardiovascular conditions would be assumed to portend a higher risk for cardiac arrest (Fig. 2). Furthermore, early in the pandemic, limitations in PPE and lack of rapid testing availability led to changes to emergency procedures including delaying percutaneous coronary intervention for some patients with ST segment elevation myocardial infarction.[55,56] The psychosocial

stress and reluctance to seek care in addition to the limitation of outpatient medical visits and the reduction in elective procedures are all likely contributors to the increased incidence of cardiac arrest.[11,18]

Finally, overwhelmed health care systems experienced challenges in handling the demands of hospitalized patients with COVID-19, in-hospital allocation of resources, and shortages in critical care services, including medical teams, equipment, and ICU bed availability.[6] With less available hospital resources during the pandemic, a higher threshold for hospital admission could have led to more at-risk patients for cardiac arrest being discharged from emergency departments. Response times for EMS were delayed, likely related to an overwhelmed EMS response system, emergency department overcrowding, and the need to use PPE during resuscitation.[12,51] There were also higher rates of nontransport in EMS systems, leaving patients potentially at risk for clinical deterioration.[57]

FUTURE CONSIDERATIONS
Cardiac Arrest Management

Current evidence is uncertain as to whether chest compressions or defibrillation can cause aerosol generalization and increase disease transmission to providers.[58] Airway management is an aerosol-generating procedure most commonly performed by EMS during cardiac arrest resuscitation. Therefore, a careful balance is necessary between the benefits of early resuscitation and the potential for harm to health care providers during resuscitative efforts. Consensus statements from multiple committees agree that chain of survival should be maintained including bystander CPR and public access defibrillation.[58–60] Furthermore, the use of PPE is recommended to ensure the safety of health care professionals during resuscitation, although defibrillation may be considered before donning airborne PPE.

The pandemic has led some to suggest modifications to cardiac arrest care including (1) use of field point-of-care ultrasonography to assess for cardiac standstill as means to supplement prognostication[25]; (2) reduction in the duration of CPR cycle from 2 to 1 minute, given the deterioration in the quality of chest compressions among rescuers wearing PPE[61]; and (3) placement of a towel or mask over the patient's mouth and nose during cardiac resuscitation with compression-only CPR.[60] These modifications may be reasonable as long as they do not interfere with high-quality CPR.

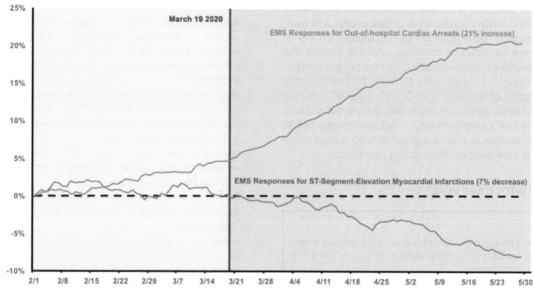

Fig. 2. Los Angeles county out-of-hospital nontraumatic cardiac arrest and ST segment elevation calls, March 19 to May 29, 2020. Significant increase in EMS calls for out-of-hospital cardiac arrest and a significant decrease in EMS call for ST segment elevation myocardial infarction in Los Angeles County, CA, USA. (*From* Rollman, J.E., et al., Emergency Medical Services Responses to Out-of-Hospital Cardiac Arrest and Suspected ST-Segment Elevation Myocardial Infarction During the COVID-19 Pandemic in Los Angeles County. J Am Heart Assoc, 2021. 10(12): p. e019635.)

Public Messaging

Particularly early in the pandemic, public health department messaging urged people to stay at home and lockdowns were implemented to reduce movement and potential exposure. Although a justifiable and important step to reduce the spread of infection, patients also avoided and minimized visits to outpatient clinics and to hospitals, likely due to this messaging as well as perceived risk of disease contagion. Studies published to date suggest that this resulted in worse outcome for time-sensitive cardiovascular medical conditions including cardiac arrest, ST segment elevation myocardial infarction, and stroke.[7] In response, multiple public messaging campaigns have been initiated.[62] Future messaging should continue to consider the impact on preventative and emergency care and to balance the concern for public and provider safety with the risk of delaying care for time-sensitive emergencies.

System-Level Pandemic Response

Many health care systems became overwhelmed with the surge of patients with acute respiratory illness and when baseline preventative health and emergency services broke down. Delays to both routine and emergency care led to increased severity of illness. Health care systems must consider how to maintain these services while responding to a pandemic surge. Many innovative programs to optimize resources were developed in response to the pandemic and can serve as models for expansion.[63] Building up telemedicine capabilities and mobile-integrated health programs can help to maintain standard medical care when access to hospital care is limited and/or public concern leads to changes in care-seeking behavior.[64] Dispatch support systems, use of advanced providers for triage, and alternate destinations for transport can optimize deployment of EMS resources to preserve rapid response for time-sensitive emergencies.

SUMMARY

During the COVID-19 pandemic both OHCA and IHCA have increased in incidence while outcomes among patients suffering cardiac arrest are worse. Direct effects of the COVID-19 illness as well as indirect effects of the pandemic on patient's behavior and health care systems have contributed to these changes. Understanding these potential factors offers the opportunity to improve future response and save lives. Fortunately, compared with the first wave of the COVID-19 pandemic, subsequent spikes in COVID-19 incidence seem to show an increase of lesser magnitude of cardiac arrest despite an overall increase in COVID-19 infections. As health care systems have adapted, experience gained from the first wave may have led to better management of patients with COVID-19, allocation of resources, and evaluation of non-COVID medical issues. Efforts at mass vaccination continue and will reduce the severity of disease leading to less severe complications for those with COVID-19. The adverse impact of delaying non-COVID medical care has become readily apparent, prompting the science and medical community to widely release public campaigns to encourage patients to pursue medical care despite the ongoing pandemic.

CLINICS CARE POINTS

- Clinicians should be aware that cardiac arrest incidence has increased during the COVID-19 pandemic.
- The chain of survival should be maintained, including bystander CPR and public access defibrillation.
- Healthcare professionals should use personal protective equipment to reduce risk of exposure during cardiac arrest resuscitation.
- It is important to maintain systems of care during respiratory pandemics in order to reduce harm of delayed access to routine and emergency care.

DISCLOSURE

There are no disclosures from any of the authors.

REFERENCES

1. Virani SS, et al. Heart disease and stroke Statistics-2020 Update: a report from the American heart association. Circulation 2020;141(9):e139–596.
2. Merchant RM, et al. Hospital variation in survival after in-hospital cardiac arrest. J Am Heart Assoc 2014;3(1):e000400.
3. Sasson C, et al. Predictors of survival from out-of-hospital cardiac arrest: a systematic review and meta-analysis. Circ Cardiovasc Qual Outcomes 2010;3(1):63–81.
4. Tracker COVID-19 World Health Organization. 2021. https://covid19.who.int/.
5. Rea T, Kudenchuk PJ. Death by COVID-19: an open investigation. J Am Heart Assoc 2021;10(12): e021764.
6. Kiss P, et al. The impact of the COVID-19 pandemic on the care and management of patients with acute cardiovascular disease: a systematic review. Eur Heart J Qual Care Clin Outcomes 2021;7(1):18–27.
7. Rollman JE, et al. Emergency medical services responses to out-of-hospital cardiac arrest and suspected ST-segment-elevation myocardial infarction during the COVID-19 pandemic in Los Angeles county. J Am Heart Assoc 2021;10(12): e019635.
8. Marijon E, et al. Out-of-hospital cardiac arrest during the COVID-19 pandemic in Paris, France: a population-based, observational study. Lancet Public Health 2020;5(8):e437–43.
9. Mathew S, et al. Effects of the COVID-19 pandemic on out-of-hospital cardiac arrest care in Detroit. Am J Emerg Med 2021;46:90–6.
10. Baldi E, et al. Out-of-Hospital cardiac arrest during the covid-19 outbreak in Italy. N Engl J Med 2020; 383(5):496–8.
11. Huber BC, et al. Out-of-hospital cardiac arrest incidence during COVID-19 pandemic in Southern Germany. Resuscitation 2020;157:121–2.
12. Lai PH, et al. Characteristics associated with out-of-hospital cardiac arrests and resuscitations during the novel coronavirus disease 2019 pandemic in New York city. JAMA Cardiol 2020;5(10):1154–63.
13. Lim SL, et al. Incidence and outcomes of out-of-hospital cardiac arrest in Singapore and Victoria: a Collaborative study. J Am Heart Assoc 2020;9(21): e015981.
14. Paoli A, et al. Out-of-hospital cardiac arrest during the COVID-19 pandemic in the Province of Padua, Northeast Italy. Resuscitation 2020;154:47–9.
15. Elmer J, et al. Indirect effects of COVID-19 on OHCA in a low prevalence region. Resuscitation 2020;156: 282–3.
16. Sayre MR, et al. Prevalence of COVID-19 in out-of-hospital cardiac arrest: implications for bystander cardiopulmonary resuscitation. Circulation 2020; 142(5):507–9.
17. Chan PS, et al. Outcomes for out-of-hospital cardiac arrest in the United States during the coronavirus disease 2019 pandemic. JAMA Cardiol 2021;6(3): 296–303.
18. Marijon E, Karam N, Jouven X. Cardiac arrest occurrence during successive waves of the COVID-19 pandemic: direct and indirect consequences. Eur Heart J 2021;42(11):1107–9.
19. Sultanian P, et al. Cardiac arrest in COVID-19: characteristics and outcomes of in- and out-of-hospital cardiac arrest. A report from the Swedish Registry for Cardiopulmonary Resuscitation. Eur Heart J 2021;42(11):1094–106.
20. Scquizzato T, et al. Effects of COVID-19 pandemic on out-of-hospital cardiac arrests: a systematic review. Resuscitation 2020;157:241–7.
21. Lim ZJ, et al. Incidence and outcome of out-of-hospital cardiac arrests in the COVID-19 era: a systematic review and meta-analysis. Resuscitation 2020;157:248–58.

22. Yu JH, et al. Impact of the COVID-19 pandemic on emergency medical service response to out-of-hospital cardiac arrests in Taiwan: a retrospective observational study. Emerg Med J 2021;38(9):679–84.

23. Lim D, et al. The comparison of emergency medical service responses to and outcomes of out-of-hospital cardiac arrest before and during the COVID-19 pandemic in an area of Korea. J Korean Med Sci 2021;36(36):e255.

24. Abrahamson SD, Canzian S, Brunet F. Using simulation for training and to change protocol during the outbreak of severe acute respiratory syndrome. Crit Care 2006;10(1):R3.

25. Ong J, et al. An international perspective of out-of-hospital cardiac arrest and cardiopulmonary resuscitation during the COVID-19 pandemic. Am J Emerg Med 2021;47:192–7.

26. Edelson DP, et al. Interim Guidance for basic and advanced life support in Adults, Children, and Neonates with suspected or confirmed COVID-19: from the emergency cardiovascular care committee and Get with the guidelines-resuscitation adult and Pediatric task forces of the American heart association. Circulation 2020;141(25):e933–43.

27. Morrison LJ, et al. Strategies for improving survival after in-hospital cardiac arrest in the United States: 2013 consensus recommendations: a consensus statement from the American Heart Association. Circulation 2013;127(14):1538–63.

28. Andersen LW, et al. In-hospital cardiac arrest: a review. JAMA 2019;321(12):1200–10.

29. Shao F, et al. In-hospital cardiac arrest outcomes among patients with COVID-19 pneumonia in Wuhan, China. Resuscitation 2020;151:18–23.

30. Aldabagh M, et al. Survival of in-hospital cardiac arrest in COVID-19 infected patients. Healthcare (Basel) 2021;9(10).

31. Miles JA, et al. Characteristics and outcomes of in-hospital cardiac arrest events during the COVID-19 pandemic: a Single-Center experience from a New York city public hospital. Circ Cardiovasc Qual Outcomes 2020;13(11):e007303.

32. Hayek SS, et al. In-hospital cardiac arrest in critically ill patients with covid-19: multicenter cohort study. BMJ 2020;371:m3513.

33. Roedl K, et al. Effects of COVID-19 on in-hospital cardiac arrest: incidence, causes, and outcome - a retrospective cohort study. Scand J Trauma Resusc Emerg Med 2021;29(1):30.

34. Tong SK, et al. Effect of the COVID-19 pandemic on cardiac arrest resuscitation practices and outcomes in non-COVID-19 patients. J Intensive Care 2021;9(1):55.

35. Chelly J, et al. OHCA (Out-of-Hospital cardiac arrest) and CAHP (cardiac arrest hospital prognosis) scores to predict outcome after in-hospital cardiac arrest: Insight from a multicentric registry. Resuscitation 2020;156:167–73.

36. Thapa SB, et al. Clinical outcomes of in-hospital cardiac arrest in COVID-19. JAMA Intern Med 2021;181(2):279–81.

37. Worku E, et al. Provision of ECPR during COVID-19: evidence, equity, and ethical dilemmas. Crit Care 2020;24(1):462.

38. Douma MJ, Mackenzie E, Brindley PG, et al. A novel and cost-free solution to ensuring adequate chest compressions. Resuscitation 2020;152:93–4.

39. Poole K, et al. Mechanical CPR: who? When? How? Crit Care 2018;22(1):140.

40. Shaefi S, et al. Extracorporeal membrane oxygenation in patients with severe respiratory failure from COVID-19. Intensive Care Med 2021;47(2):208–21.

41. Ippolito M, et al. Mortality after in-hospital cardiac arrest in patients with COVID-19: a systematic review and meta-analysis. Resuscitation 2021;164:122–9.

42. Mahase E, Kmietowicz Z. Covid-19: Doctors are told not to perform CPR on patients in cardiac arrest. BMJ 2020;368:m1282.

43. Rubins JB, Kinzie SD, Rubins DM. Predicting outcomes of in-hospital cardiac arrest: retrospective US validation of the Good outcome following attempted resuscitation Score. J Gen Intern Med 2019;34(11):2530–5.

44. Libby P, Luscher T. COVID-19 is, in the end, an endothelial disease. Eur Heart J 2020;41(32):3038–44.

45. Fried JA, et al. The variety of cardiovascular presentations of COVID-19. Circulation 2020;141(23):1930–6.

46. Madjid M, et al. Potential effects of Coronaviruses on the cardiovascular system: a review. JAMA Cardiol 2020;5(7):831–40.

47. Fauvel C, et al. Pulmonary embolism in COVID-19 patients: a French multicentre cohort study. Eur Heart J 2020;41(32):3058–68.

48. Klok FA, et al. Incidence of thrombotic complications in critically ill ICU patients with COVID-19. Thromb Res 2020;191:145–7.

49. Mercuro NJ, et al. Risk of QT interval Prolongation associated with Use of hydroxychloroquine with or without concomitant azithromycin among hospitalized patients testing positive for coronavirus disease 2019 (COVID-19). JAMA Cardiol 2020;5(9):1036–41.

50. Ball J, et al. Collateral damage: Hidden impact of the COVID-19 pandemic on the out-of-hospital cardiac arrest system-of-care. Resuscitation 2020;156:157–63.

51. Baldi E, et al. COVID-19 kills at home: the close relationship between the epidemic and the increase of out-of-hospital cardiac arrests. Eur Heart J 2020;41(32):3045–54.

52. Holt-Lunstad J, et al. Loneliness and social isolation as risk factors for mortality: a meta-analytic review. Perspect Psychol Sci 2015;10(2):227–37.

53. Friedman J, Akre S. COVID-19 and the drug overdose Crisis: Uncovering the Deadliest Months in the United States, January-July 2020. Am J Public Health 2021;111(7):1284–91.

54. Gluckman TJ, et al. Case rates, treatment approaches, and outcomes in acute myocardial infarction during the coronavirus disease 2019 pandemic. JAMA Cardiol 2020;5(12):1419–24.

55. Jain V, et al. Management of STEMI during the COVID-19 pandemic: Lessons learned in 2020 to prepare for 2021. Trends Cardiovasc Med 2021; 31(3):135–40.

56. Hakim R, Motreff P, Range G. [COVID-19 and STEMI]. Ann Cardiol Angeiol (Paris) 2020;69(6): 355–9.

57. Harrison NE, et al. Factors associated with Voluntary Refusal of emergency medical system transport for emergency care in Detroit during the early Phase of the COVID-19 pandemic. JAMA Netw Open 2021;4(8):e2120728.

58. Perkins GD, et al. International Liaison Committee on Resuscitation: COVID-19 consensus on science, treatment recommendations and task force insights. Resuscitation 2020;151:145–7.

59. Nolan JP, et al. European Resuscitation Council COVID-19 guidelines executive summary. Resuscitation 2020;153:45–55.

60. Craig S, et al. Management of adult cardiac arrest in the COVID-19 era: consensus statement from the Australasian College for Emergency Medicine. Med J Aust 2020;213(3):126–33.

61. Malysz M, et al. An optimal chest compression technique using personal protective equipment during resuscitation in the COVID-19 pandemic: a randomized crossover simulation study. Kardiol Pol 2020; 78(12):1254–61.

62. Caltabellotta T, et al. Characteristics associated with patient delay during the management of ST-segment elevated myocardial infarction, and the influence of awareness campaigns. Arch Cardiovasc Dis 2021; 114(4):305–15.

63. Monaghesh E, Hajizadeh A. The role of telehealth during COVID-19 outbreak: a systematic review based on current evidence. BMC Public Health 2020;20(1):1193.

64. Demeke HB, et al. Trends in Use of telehealth among health centers during the COVID-19 pandemic - United States, June 26-November 6, 2020. MMWR Morb Mortal Wkly Rep 2021;70(7):240–4.

Mechanical Complication of Acute Myocardial Infarction Secondary to COVID-19 Disease

Abdulla A. Damluji, MD, PhD, MPH[a,b,*], Nikhil R. Gangasani, MPH[c,d], Cindy L. Grines, MD[c,d]

KEYWORDS

- COVID-19 • Mechanical Complications • Reperfusion therapies • Myocardial infarction
- Cardiogenic shock

KEY POINTS

- The COVID-19 pandemic has led to an increase in mechanical complications of AMI. The outcomes for these complications are poor without a prompt recognition and a systematic approach to management.
- Mechanical complications during the COVID-19 pandemic were mostly due to delayed presentation after AMI in the context of "stay-at-home" orders, mandating that all residents stay home unless they hold an essential job or have an essential need for daily living.
- The most commonly encountered mechanical complications are ventricular septal defect, papillary muscle rupture, free wall rupture, and pseudoaneurysm.
- The approach to management of these complications includes a high level of suspicion, especially in patients with severe hemodynamic changes and pulmonary congestion after a presentation with an acute myocardial infarction.
- The involvement of "Heart Team" provides a systematic platform to discuss all therapeutic options for hemodynamic support, oxygenation status, percutaneous or surgical repair, and end of life care in the CICU.
- To provide a comprehensive team-based approach to management, the multidisciplinary heart teams should ideally include a cardiac intensivist, cardiac surgeon, interventional cardiologist, imaging specialist, transplant specialist, respiratory therapist, clinical pharmacist, family members, and palliative care teams.

INTRODUCTION

The aggressive inflammatory response to COVID-19 can result in airway damage, respiratory failure, cardiac injury, and multiorgan failure, which lead to death in susceptible patients.[1,2] Cardiac injury and acute myocardial infarction (AMI) secondary to

This article originally appeared in Cardiology Clinics, Volume 40, Issue 3, August 2022.
Presentation: None.
Funding and Financial Disclosure: Dr A.A. Damluji receives research funding from the Pepper Scholars Program of the Johns Hopkins University Claude D. Pepper Older Americans Independence Center funded by the National Institute on Aging P30-AG021334 and Dr A.A. Damluji receives mentored patient-oriented research career development award from the National Heart, Lung, and Blood Institute K23-HL153771-01.
[a] Johns Hopkins University School of Medicine, 1800 Orleans Street, Baltimore, MD 21287, USA; [b] Inova Center of Outcomes Research, 3300 Gallows Road, Falls Church, VA 22042, USA; [c] Medical College of Georgia, 1120 15th Street, Augusta, GA 30912, USA; [d] Northside Hospital Cardiovascular Institute, 1000 Johnson Ferry Road NorthEast, GA 30041, USA
* Corresponding author. Inova Center of Outcomes Research, 3300 Gallows Road, Falls Church, VA 22042.
E-mail address: Abdulla.Damluji@jhu.edu

COVID-19 disease can lead to hospitalization, heart failure, and sudden cardiac death.[3] When serious collateral damage from tissue necrosis or bleeding occurs, mechanical complications of myocardial infarction and cardiogenic shock can ensue. While prompt reperfusion therapies have decreased the incidence of these serious complications, patients who present late following the initial infarct are at increased for mechanical complications, cardiogenic shock, and death. The health outcomes for patients with mechanical complications are dismal if not recognized and treated promptly.[4] Even if they survive serious pump failure, their CICU stay is often prolonged, and their index hospitalization and follow-up visits may consume significant resources and impact the health care system.[4]

After the spread of the COVID-19 in the United States and the world, an increase in the incidence of mechanical complications of AMI was observed, likely because of delayed presentation in patients without COVID-19.[4–8] Cardiologists, cardiac intensivists, and surgeons are faced with the challenges of managing mechanical complications and the associated discussion on appropriate therapies often occurs among heart teams in specialized shock centers. Prompt recognition of clinical signs and symptoms of acute pump failure is needed to avoid prolonged states of shock, advanced forms of heart failure, and death. Differentiation between mechanical complications of type I and type II AMI secondary to COVID-19 infection requires clinical bedside knowledge, utilization of noninvasive imaging, and invasive hemodynamic assessment. Even if the diagnosis is made promptly, the management of these patients is often complex and requires the expertise of multidisciplinary teams. Because post-MI mechanical defects are rare, the management is variable depending on the expertise of each cardiac center caring for these patients. This article aims to address the most common mechanical complications encountered after COVID-19 disease; (2) define a multidisciplinary approach to management; and (3) highlight a case series discussing management strategies in practice.

VENTRICULAR SEPTAL DEFECT

Before thrombolysis and primary revascularization became the standard of care, the incidence of ventricular septal defects (VSD) caused by transmural myocardial infarct rupture was approximately 1% to 2%, compared with less than 0.3% in contemporary practice.[4] Risk factors include older age, female sex, and delayed reperfusion.[4] Typically occurring 3 to 5 days postinfarction, presentations range from incidental findings to circulatory collapse. Symptoms may include recurrent chest pain, dyspnea, and orthopnea. Clinical examination may reveal a systolic murmur, rales, hypotension, cool skin, with signs of pulmonary venous congestion.[4] A 12-lead electrocardiogram may identify progressive ischemia and associated arrythmias.[4]

Echocardiography is diagnostic, evaluating size and location of a left-to-right shunt (**Fig. 1**), biventricular function, presence of LV thrombus, mitral regurgitation, pulmonary artery and right-sided pressures, free-wall rupture and tamponade.[4] Right heart catheterization shows a diagnostic step-up in oxygenation between the right atrium and pulmonary artery and elevated pulmonary-to-systemic flow ratio (up to 8:1) depending on the ventricular septal defect (VSD) size.[4] Left heart catheterization commonly shows a complete coronary obstruction without collateral circulation and left ventriculography shows contrast in the right ventricle and pulmonary artery.[4] Anterior and apical ischemic VSDs are caused by infarcts in the left anterior descending (LAD) territory and posterior VSDs are due to inferior infarcts.[4] Right ventricular infarction or ischemia with severe dysfunction is an important feature of VSDs caused by acute, proximal right coronary occlusion.[4] Posterior VSDs are often accompanied by mitral valve regurgitation commonly secondary to ischemic remodeling.[4]

Because of the 80% 30-day mortality associated with uncorrected defects, medical therapy alone is limited to hemodynamically insignificant defects, or prohibitive risk patients.[4] Effective afterload reduction to decrease the left-to-right shunt is essential: intra-aortic balloon pumps or impella with pharmacotherapy are used in more than 80% of emergencies and 65% of urgent repairs. Temporary percutaneous ventricular assist devices are increasingly used.[4] Patients severely compromised by multi-organ failure may benefit from biventricular mechanical support or extracorporal membrane oxygenation with percutaneous or surgical left ventricular vents, allowing end-organ recovery before definitive surgery.[4] Emergency surgery is indicated for cardiogenic shock with pulmonary edema refractory to mechanical circulatory support. Lower mortality is reported when surgery is delayed for a week after diagnosis, although selection and survival bias may explain this.

Coronary bypasses are performed first, commonly with saphenous veins, to facilitate myocardial protection and minimize handling of the heart after VSD repair. Primary repair (Dagett) or infarct exclusion (David) techniques are used.[4] For anterior VSDs the infarcted surface of the

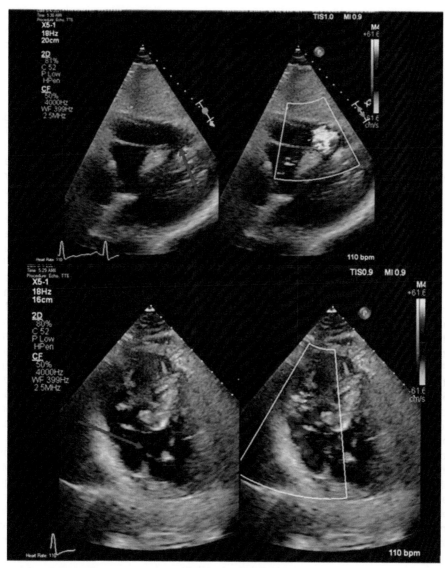

Fig. 1. Ventricular septal defect with left-to-right shunting (*red arrow*).

anterolateral left ventricle (LV) is incised parallel to the LAD.[4] The defect in the septum is usually immediately beneath the incision. A patch repair using pericardium is performed using mattress sutures with the pledgets on the right ventricular side in noninfarcted myocardium, so the whole LV aspect of the septum is excluded from the mitral annulus to the anterolateral LV wall.[4] It is usually possible to close the left ventriculotomy primarily with mattress sutures buttressed with pericardium or felt, reinforced with continuous sutures and bioglue. True apical VSDs can be repaired and closed primarily by amputating the apex.[4] Posterior VSDs are approached via a ventriculotomy in the infarcted posterior LV wall parallel to the posterior descending coronary artery, attaching a patch to

the LV aspect of the noninfarcted septum with patch closure, primary closure or infarct exclusion depending on how much free ventricular wall is infarcted.[4] Temporary left ventricular assist devices to decompress the LV reducing the risk of left ventriculotomy rupture and supporting cardiac output postoperatively. The 40% perioperative mortality has not changed significantly in decades.[1,4] There have been case reports and small series of percutaneous VSD closure using PFO closure devices, with variable outcomes.

Ventricular Septal Defects Case

A 50-year-old Hispanic male developed chest pain radiating to the back greater than 72 hours before

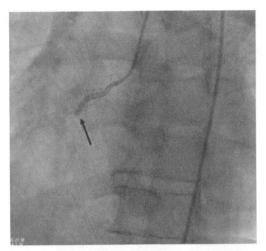

Fig. 2. Coronary angiogram demonstrating 100% occlusion of the right coronary artery (*red arrow*).

admission. He reported a similar self-limiting episode a week prior. He presented to the hospital whereby he was found to be in Killip class 4 heart failure and inferior MI. His initial heart rate was 123 BPM, BP 74/56. He was COVID-19 negative. Emergent cardiac catheterization revealed 3 vessel coronary disease with 100% occlusion of the right coronary (**Fig. 2**) and LAD with no collaterals. Placement of 4 stents in the mid and distal right coronary failed to restore flow and remained TIMI 0. Echocardiography performed during catheterization showed EF greater than 70% and inferior apical VSD (**Fig. 3**). The patient was ultimately maintained on an intra-aortic balloon pump and transferred to a quaternary care facility whereby he underwent surgical repair, had impella and ECMO placed but ultimately expired.

Case 2

A 74-year-old Caucasian female developed chest pain after receiving her COVID-19 shot 1 week before admission but did not seek medical attention. She later presented to the hospital whereby she was found to be in Killip class 4 heart failure and ECG showing anterior MI. Her initial heart rate was 122 BPM, BP 103/73. She was COVID-19 negative. Emergent cardiac catheterization demonstrated 2 vessel coronary diseases with 100% occlusion of the proximal left anterior descending (**Fig. 4**) with no collaterals. She underwent placement of a stent that restored TIMI-3 flow. After catheterization, left ventriculography showed the presence of a ventricular septal defect (**Fig. 5**). EF was estimated at 15% to 20%. The patient was ultimately maintained on an intra-aortic balloon pump and transferred to a quaternary

care facility. She underwent VSD repair 10 days later but decompensated and died 3 weeks after initial hospital presentation despite support with ECMO and renal replacement therapy.

PAPILLARY MUSCLE RUPTURE

The incidence of acute severe mitral regurgitation (**Fig. 6**) from papillary muscle rupture (PMR), like other mechanical complications of acute MI (AMI), has declined in the reperfusion era to less than 0.05%.[4] Primary PCI has further reduced the incidence compared with thrombolysis. Despite this decline, excess hospital mortality is reported compared with patients with AMI without PMR (36.3% vs 5.3%) in the current era.[1]

PMR occurs most frequently after inferior AMI in patients with no history of prior CAD. It is more common with STEMI than NSTEMI. The posteromedial papillary muscle is more often involved because of its single blood supply.[4] PMR may be complete or partial, which may affect the ease of diagnosis and severity of clinical symptoms.[4] Risk factors for PMR include older age, lack of revascularization after AMI, and delay in presentation after AMI.[2] PMR typically occurs within 7 days of AMI.[4] Patients present with pulmonary edema and may quickly progress to cardiogenic shock (CS). A murmur may be absent due to the equalization of left atrial and left ventricular pressures. Transthoracic echocardiography may not be diagnostic, particularly in cases of partial PMR. Transesophageal echocardiography or angiographic left ventriculography (**Fig. 7**) has a high diagnostic sensitivity.[4] Left ventricular ejection fraction is often normal or low-normal. Coronary angiography will most often demonstrate single or 2-vessel CAD, with total occlusion of the infarct-related artery.

Patients may require mechanical ventilation. A pulmonary artery catheter is useful for the titration of vasoactive medications. Patients that do not present with CS commonly experience rapid deterioration of their hemodynamics. An intra-aortic balloon pump may be beneficial for patients with CS and the experience with mechanical circulatory support, including percutaneous VADs and VA-ECMO for stabilization in PMR is limited. Emergent mitral valve surgery is the standard treatment, and it should occur within hours of diagnosis. For patients that are hemodynamically stable on support, the urgency of mitral valve surgery may be diminished.

Patients included in the surgical series of PMR treatment are highly selected and their outcomes cannot be generalized to all-comers.[4] Many patients with PMR are not offered surgery. In the

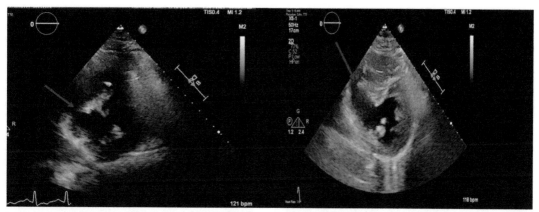

Fig. 3. Arrow shows the inferior apical ventricular septal defect.

SHOCK trial registry, only 38% of patients with CS from acute severe MR after AMI were offered mitral valve surgery.[3] A recent analysis of AMI admissions from the National Inpatient Sample found that only 58% of patients with PMR underwent mitral valve surgery.[1] Factors that may influence this decision include advanced age, comorbidities, and inability to stabilize the patient while awaiting surgery.[4]

Chordal-sparing mitral valve replacement is generally preferred over repair because the operation is predictable and its durability established. Small series have reported repair techniques, typically for patients with partial PMR and less preoperative hemodynamic derangement.[4] Concomitant CABG should be considered in patients with PMR and severe CAD. The surgeon must weigh the risks and benefits of prolonging the operation with CABG. Some surgical series have reported improved outcomes with concomitant CABG. Recently there have been reports of using percutaneous mitral clip repairs with reasonable results.[4]

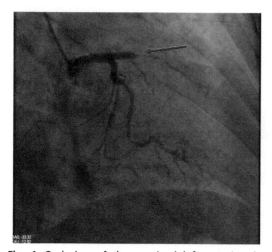

Fig. 4. Occlusion of the proximal left anterior descending artery (*red arrow*).

Papillary Muscle Rupture Case

A 60-year-old Caucasian male developed chest pain greater than 72 hours before admission. Due to progressive dyspnea, he presented to the hospital whereby he was found to be in Killip class 3 heart failure. His initial heart rate was 116 BPM, BP 90/62 mm Hg, pulmonary rales and systolic murmur were noted. He was COVID-19 negative. Emergent cardiac catheterization demonstrated 3 vessel coronary disease with 100% occlusion of the circumflex with no collaterals. He underwent placement of 4 stents in the circumflex, second obtuse marginal branch, and left main coronary with the restoration of TIMI 3 flow. After catheterization, echocardiography showed EF of 35% to 40% with posterior papillary muscle rupture (**Fig. 8**). The patient was scheduled for surgical mitral valve repair but developed sudden cardiogenic shock and died 4 days after hospital presentation.

FREE WALL RUPTURE

Although free wall rupture (FWR) is the most common mechanical complication following acute myocardial infarction, its true incidence is unknown because of out of hospital sudden cardiac death and lack of routine autopsy.[4] While the overall incidence of rupture has undoubtedly decreased with prompt acute reperfusion therapy for STEMI, the early hazard noted at 24 hours in thrombolytic versus placebo trials established the risk of FWR with delayed reperfusion therapy.[4,9] This phenomenon is attributed to intramyocardial hemorrhage, myocardial dissection, and subsequent rupture: a phenomenon that has also been noted following primary percutaneous intervention.[4,10]

Free wall rupture should be suspected in any patient with hemodynamic instability or collapse following an AMI, especially in the setting of

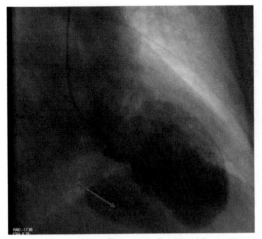

Fig. 5. Left ventriculography shows contrast in both left and right ventricles, demonstrating ventricular septal defect (*red arrow*).

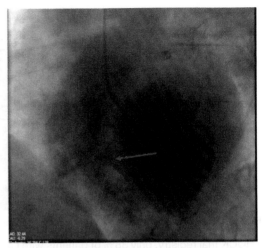

Fig. 7. Arrow indicates ventricular septal defect on left ventriculography.

delayed, ineffective, or absent reperfusion therapy.[4] The clinical examination classically shows jugular venous distension, a pulsus paradoxus or frank electromechanical disassociation and muffled heart sounds in the setting of cardiovascular collapse.[4] It is sometimes preceded by chest pain and nausea, and EKG may show new ST elevation as contact with blood irritates the pericardium. Instant death is common in a blowout rupture, but in exceptional cases, a prompt bedside echocardiogram confirms the diagnosis and warrants emergent surgical correction. A variant of frank rupture characterized by a mushy infarct zone with an oozing bloody pericardial effusion should be recognized.[4] In cases of circulatory collapse, immediate placement on ECMO support may provide an opportunity to stabilize the circulation and perform the definitive repair with acceptable results.[4,11]

The initial surgical repair was performed by Fitzgibbons and involved an infarctectomy with defect closure on cardiopulmonary bypass.[4,12] The goals of surgical intervention revolve around repairing the defect, treating tamponade, and leaving behind adequate healthy tissue that will minimize late complications.[4,13] The preferred technique used is guided by anatomy and presentation, and may rarely be limited to a linear closure, but often involves an infarctectomy when extensive necrosis is present with patch closure with materials such as Dacron or pericardium. The ideal repair when anatomy allows is a primary patch repair that covers the defect but when feasible a sutureless repair using a patch and glue or a collagen sponge patch can be performed with or without the need for ongoing cardiopulmonary bypass. A percutaneous approach using intra pericardial fibrin-glue injection is evolving.[4]

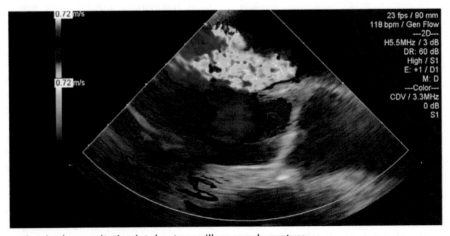

Fig. 6. Eccentric mitral regurgitation jet due to papillary muscle rupture.

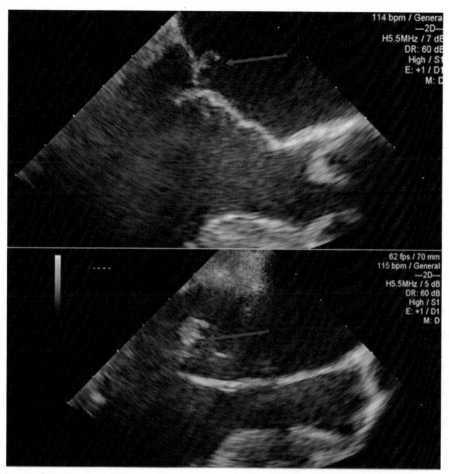

Fig. 8. Evidence of ruptured posterior papillary muscle on echocardiography (*red arrow*).

PSEUDOANEURYSM

Pseudoaneurysms of the left ventricle develop when cardiac rupture is contained by pericardial adhesions.[4,14–18] Although they may occur following cardiovascular surgery, blunt or penetrating chest trauma, or as a result of infective endocarditis, they are most commonly associated with prior acute myocardial infarction.[4,15–18] Compared with true aneurysms, pseudoaneurysms more often involve the posterior or lateral wall—perhaps the result of dependent pericardial adhesions developing in the recumbent, convalescing postinfarction patient.[4] While acute anterior wall rupture is thought to result in unrelenting hemopericardium, catastrophic tamponade, and immediate death, other pseudoaneurysms can remain undiagnosed for several months or longer.[4,15–18]

Patients with pseudoaneurysm may present with a myriad of signs or symptoms, none of which can be considered pathognomonic for the condition. While previous case series have argued that nearly half of afflicted individuals will be asymptomatic at the time of diagnosis,[18] more contemporary studies and systematic reviews instead note that the majority will be expected to present with congestive heart failure, chest pain, or shortness of breath. Others may develop symptomatic arrhythmias, signs of systemic embolization, and even sudden cardiac death. Most patients are male, and will have both electrocardiographic (eg, ST-segment changes) and radiographic (eg, "mass-like" protuberance on plain film or cardiomegaly) abnormalities at presentation.[4,14] Diagnosis requires a high index of suspicion and often necessitates the use of multiple complimentary imaging tools; among these include coronary angiography and ventriculography, two-dimensional transthoracic echocardiography, transesophageal echocardiography, cardiac computed tomography, and magnetic resonance imaging.[11–15] Pseudoaneurysms will usually have a narrow neck and, as noted above, will lack the normal structural elements found in an intact cardiac wall.[4]

Left ventricular pseudoaneurysms are felt to represent surgical emergencies due to their high risk for progressive rupture. In truth, however, little is known about the natural history of medically managed disease. In one small series of patients at the Mayo Clinic, none of those treated conservatively (without operative intervention) succumbed to fatal hemorrhage. Instead, the majority died as a result of other complications, including recurrent ischemia or progressive heart failure.[14] It is important to acknowledge that the contemporary literature is quite sparse, and likely undermined by selection and publication bias. While case reports of percutaneous repair exist,[15] most experts still believe that immediate surgical management is prudent. Surgeons should be prepared to quickly institute cardiopulmonary bypass at the time of operative intervention, as rupture and hemodynamic collapse can occur soon after pericardial manipulation.[4]

SUMMARY

COVID-19 disease resulted in a substantial increase in the incidence of myocardial injury, heart failure, and death. In addition, stay-at-home mandates and patient fear of contracting COVID-19 at the hospital has the unintended consequence of fewer patients with STEMI being treated. In severe cases, mechanical complication of AMI can occur particularly among those with delayed presentation after initial cardiac injury. Without a prompt and systematic approach to management, the outcomes for patients with mechanical complications are poor. The management involves a high level of suspicion, particularly among patients with hemodynamic compromise. The utilization of "Heart Team" facilitates a systematic approach to management and ensures a discussion of all therapeutic options to provide hemodynamic stability and durable outcomes.

CLINICS CARE POINTS

- The COVID-19 pandemic resulted in a higher proportion of patients with delayed presentation of myocardial infarction, which ultimately led to an increase in the incidence of mechanical complications in the U.S. and around the world.
- Prompt and systematic approach to management is needed to avoid poor outcomes. The management involves a high level of suspicion, particularly among patients with hemodynamic compromise. The utilization of "Heart Team" facilitates a systematic approach to management and ensures a

discussion of all therapeutic options to provide hemodynamic stability and durable outcomes.

ACKNOWLEDGMENTS

None.

DISCLOSURE

The authors have nothing to disclose.

REFERENCES

1. Fauci AS, Lane HC, Redfield RR. Covid-19 - navigating the uncharted. N Engl J Med 2020;382(13):1268–9.
2. Damluji AA, Wei S, Bruce SA, et al. Seropositivity of COVID-19 among asymptomatic healthcare workers: a multi-site prospective cohort study from Northern Virginia, United States. Lancet Reg Health Am 2021;2:100030.
3. Rosner CM, Genovese L, Tehrani BN, et al. Myocarditis Temporally associated with COVID-19 Vaccination. Circulation 2021;144(6):502–5.
4. Alsidawi S, Campbell A, Tamene A, et al. Ventricular septal rupture complicating delayed acute myocardial infarction presentation during the COVID-19 Pandemic. JACC Case Rep 2020;2(10):1595–8.
5. Albiero R, Seresini G. Subacute left ventricular free wall rupture after delayed STEMI presentation during the COVID-19 Pandemic. JACC Case Rep 2020;2(10):1603–9.
6. Moroni F, Gramegna M, Ajello S, et al. Collateral damage: medical care avoidance Behavior among patients with myocardial infarction during the COVID-19 Pandemic. JACC Case Rep 2020;2(10):1620–4.
7. Damluji AA, van Diepen S, Katz JN, et al. Mechanical complications of acute myocardial infarction: a Scientific Statement from the American Heart Association. Circulation 2021;144(2):e16–35.
8. O'Gara PT, Kushner FG, Ascheim DD, et al. 2013 ACCF/AHA guideline for the management of ST-elevation myocardial infarction: a report of the American College of Cardiology Foundation/American Heart Association Task Force on practice Guidelines. Circulation 2013;127(4):e362–425.
9. Honda S, Asaumi Y, Yamane T, et al. Trends in the clinical and pathological characteristics of cardiac rupture in patients with acute myocardial infarction over 35 years. J Am Heart Assoc 2014;3(5):e000984.
10. Formica F, Mariani S, Singh G, et al. Postinfarction left ventricular free wall rupture: a 17-year single-centre experience. Eur J Cardiothorac Surg 2018;53(1):150–6.
11. FitzGibbon GM, Hooper GD, Heggtveit HA. Successful surgical treatment of postinfarction external

cardiac rupture. J Thorac Cardiovasc Surg 1972; 63(4):622–30.

12. Matteucci M, Fina D, Jiritano F, et al. Treatment strategies for post-infarction left ventricular free-wall rupture. Eur Heart J Acute Cardiovasc Care 2019; 8(4):379–87.

13. Damluji AA, Forman DE, van Diepen S, et al. Older Adults in the cardiac intensive care unit: Factoring Geriatric Syndromes in the management, Prognosis, and Process of care: a Scientific Statement from the American Heart Association. Circulation 2020; 141(2):e6–32.

14. Dudiy Y, Jelnin V, Einhorn BN, et al. Percutaneous closure of left ventricular pseudoaneurysm. Circ Cardiovasc Interv 2011;4(4):322–6.

15. Inayat F, Ghani AR, Riaz I, et al. Left ventricular pseudoaneurysm: an Overview of diagnosis and management. J Investig Med High Impact Case Rep 2018;6. 2324709618792025.

16. Mackenzie JW, Lemole GM. Pseudoaneurysm of the left ventricle. Tex Heart Inst J 1994;21(4):296–301.

17. Yeo TC, Malouf JF, Oh JK, et al. Clinical profile and outcome in 52 patients with cardiac pseudoaneurysm. Ann Intern Med 1998;128(4):299–305.

18. Prifti E, Bonacchi M, Baboci A, et al. Surgical treatment of post-infarction left ventricular pseudoaneurysm: case series highlighting various surgical strategies. Ann Med Surg (Lond) 2017;16:44–51.

Myocarditis Following COVID-19 Vaccination

Constantin A. Marschner, MD[a,b], Kirsten E. Shaw, MD[c], Felipe Sanchez Tijmes, MD[a,d], Matteo Fronza, MD[a], Sharmila Khullar, MD[e,f], Michael A. Seidman, MD, PhD[e,f], Paaladinesh Thavendiranathan, MD, SM[a,g], Jacob A. Udell, MD, MPH[g,h], Rachel M. Wald, MD[a,i], Kate Hanneman, MD, MPH[a,*]

KEYWORDS

• COVID-19 • Myocarditis • Vaccine • mRNA vaccine • Cardiac MRI

KEY POINTS

- Myocarditis following messenger RNA–based COVID-19 vaccines is rare; however, adolescent and young adult men are at highest risk.
- Chest pain is the most common symptom, with typical onset within a few days of vaccine administration.
- Cardiac MRI plays an important role in the diagnosis of acute myocarditis following vaccination, with typical findings of subepicardial late gadolinium enhancement and co-localizing edema at the basal inferior lateral wall.
- The disease course of myocarditis following COVID-19 vaccination is typically transient and mild, with resolution of symptoms within 1 to 3 weeks in most patients.
- However, longer term follow-up is needed to determine whether imaging abnormalities persist, to evaluate for adverse outcomes, and to understand the risk associated with subsequent vaccination.

INTRODUCTION

Following the discovery of severe acute respiratory syndrome coronavirus-2 (SARS-CoV-2) in December 2019, there has been intense focus on the development of vaccines to limit the contagion and severity of coronavirus disease 2019 (COVID-19). On December 11, 2020, the US Food and Drug Administration (FDA) issued emergency use authorization for the Pfizer-BioNTech COVID-19 vaccine (BNT162b2 mRNA). Since then, the FDA has approved the Pfizer-BioNTech COVID-19

This article originally appeared in Cardiology Clinics, Volume 40, Issue 3, August 2022.

[a] Department of Medical Imaging, Toronto General Hospital, Peter Munk Cardiac Center, University Health Network (UHN), University of Toronto, 1 PMB-298, 585 University Avenue, Toronto, Ontario M5G 2N2, Canada; [b] Department of Radiology, University Hospital, LMU Munich, Munich 81377, Germany; [c] Department of Graduate Medical Education, Abbott Northwestern Hospital, 800 East 28th Street, Minneapolis, MN 55407, USA; [d] Department of Medical Imaging, Clinica Santa Maria, Universidad de los Andes, Santa Maria 500, Santiago, Chile 7520378; [e] Department of Laboratory Medicine & Pathobiology, University of Toronto, 585 University Avenue, Toronto, ON M5G 2N2, Canada; [f] Laboratory Medicine Program, University Health Network, 200 Elizabeth Street, 11E-444, Toronto, Ontario M5G 2C4, Canada; [g] Division of Cardiology, Peter Munk Cardiac Centre, Toronto General Hospital, University Health Network (UHN), University of Toronto, 4N-490, 585 University Avenue, Toronto, Ontario M5G2N2, Canada; [h] Cardiovascular Division, Women's College Hospital, University of Toronto, 76 Grenville Street, Room 6324, Toronto, Ontario M5G2N2, Canada; [i] Division of Cardiology, Peter Munk Cardiac Centre, Toronto General Hospital, University Health Network (UHN), University of Toronto, 5N-517, 585 University Avenue, Toronto, Ontario M5G2N2, Canada

* Corresponding author. Department of Medical Imaging, Toronto General Hospital, Peter Munk Cardiac Center, University Health Network (UHN), University of Toronto, 1 PMB-298, 585 University Avenue, Toronto, Ontario M5G2N2, Canada.

E-mail address: kate.hanneman@uhn.ca

Twitter: @katehanneman (K.H.)

Heart Failure Clin 19 (2023) 251–264
https://doi.org/10.1016/j.hfc.2022.08.012
1551-7136/23/© 2022 Elsevier Inc. All rights reserved.

Abbreviations	
MRI	Magnetic resonance imaging
CMR	Cardiac magnetic resonance imaging
COVID-19	Coronavirus disease 2019

vaccine and has authorized 2 other vaccines for emergency use, Moderna (mRNA-1273) and Janssen/Johnson & Johnson (Ad26.COV2.S). The Janssen/Johnson & Johnson vaccine is an adenovirus vector vaccine, whereas the other 2 are messenger RNA (mRNA) vaccines. As of April 2022, more than 11.5 billion COVID-19 vaccine doses have been administered worldwide.

Several side effects have been reported after administration of COVID-19 vaccines, most of which are mild and self-limited. These side effects include pain at the injection site, lymphadenopathy ipsilateral to the site of injection, fever, chills, myalgias, headache, and fatigue.[1] Serious side effects have been reported in a very small proportion of individuals following COVID-19 vaccination, which include thrombosis with thrombocytopenia syndrome following administration of viral vector vaccines and myocarditis and pericarditis following administration of mRNA-based vaccines.[2–4]

Myocarditis is an inflammatory disease of the myocardium without an ischemic cause, which can be diagnosed by histologic, immunologic, and imaging criteria.[5] Pericarditis refers to nonischemic inflammation of the pericardium. The term myopericarditis is used when both the myocardium and pericardium are inflamed. Myocarditis following vaccination had been described very rarely before the introduction of COVID-19 vaccines, including following smallpox and anthrax vaccines.[6] Although rare, there has been intense interest in myocarditis following COVID-19 vaccination, particularly given the higher incidence of this adverse event in young men and concerns about the potential for long-term sequelae.

The purpose of the review is to evaluate the current literature related to myocarditis following COVID-19 vaccination, including the incidence, risk factors, clinical presentation, imaging findings, proposed pathophysiologic mechanisms, treatment, and prognosis.

Definition of Vaccine-Associated Myocarditis

There is no test or investigation that can establish causality for vaccine-associated myocarditis or pericarditis. These associations are based on a close temporal relationship between vaccine administration and the onset of symptoms, usually defined as within 14 days although ranges of up to a month have been reported in the literature.[7–10] The US Centers of Disease Control and Prevention (CDC) has established case definitions of acute myocarditis and pericarditis, including probable or confirmed acute myocarditis and probable acute pericarditis, summarized in **Table 1**.[3]

Incidence

In the United States, most of the data on the incidence of adverse events following vaccination have been gleaned from the Vaccine Adverse Events Reporting System (VAERS). As of January 7, 2022, VAERS had received 2478 reports of myocarditis and 1900 reports of pericarditis following COVID-19 vaccination.[11] Of note, the VAERS is a passive adverse event reporting system with limitations including reporting bias.

Postvaccine myocarditis has been documented worldwide, with no clear identified pattern of increased prevalence based on geographic region. Reported rates from different health care organizations across the world are similar, including large population-based studies from Israel and California.[12,13] A recent systematic review estimated that the overall incidence of myopericarditis following COVID-19 vaccination is 18 per million vaccine doses.[14] Compared with COVID-19 vaccines, the incidence of myopericarditis was higher following vaccination for small pox (132 per million vaccine doses) and did not differ significantly with the incidence of myopericarditis following influenza vaccination (1.3 per million vaccine dose) or other non-small pox vaccination (57 per million vaccine doses).[14]

Sex and age differences

The risk of myocarditis associated with mRNA-based COVID-19 vaccination is highest in men between 12 and 29 years of age following administration of the second dose.[8,12,13,15,16] As of June 2021, crude reporting rates of myocarditis following COVID-19 vaccination based on VAERS data were 40.6 cases per million second doses among men aged 12 to 29 years and 4.2 cases per million second doses among women aged 12 to 29 years.[17] The striking sex difference in adolescents and young adults has led to proposed pathophysiologic mechanisms related to sex hormones and has raised questions about the potential for underdiagnosis of myocarditis in women compared with men.[8]

Rates of myocarditis following COVID-19 vaccination are much lower in younger children between 5 and 11 years of age and adults older than 30 years.[17] As of December 19, 2021, reported rates of myocarditis based on VAERS data per 1 million doses of Pfizer-BioNTech COVID-19 vaccines administered were only 4 for men aged 5 to 11 years

Table 1
Centers for Disease Control and Prevention working case definitions for acute myocarditis and acute pericarditis

CDC Working Case Definitions		
Acute Myocarditis		**Acute Pericarditis**
Confirmed Case	**Probable Case**	**Probable Case**
Presence of ≥ 1 new or worsening of the following clinical symptoms[a] • Chest pain/pressure/discomfort • Dyspnea/shortness of breath • Palpitations • Syncope AND ≥ 1 of the following • Histopathologic confirmation of myocarditis • Elevated troponin greater than upper limit of normal and CMR findings consistent with myocarditis[b] AND • No other identifiable cause of the symptoms and findings	Presence of ≥ 1 new or worsening of the following clinical symptoms[a] • Chest pain/pressure/discomfort • Dyspnea/shortness of breath • Palpitations • Syncope AND ≥ 1 new finding of • Elevated troponin • ECG consistent with myocarditis[c] • Abnormal function or wall motion abnormality on echocardiography • CMR consistent with myocarditis[b] AND • No other identifiable cause of the symptoms and findings	Presence of ≥ 2 new or worsening of the following clinical symptoms • Acute chest pain (typically described as pain made worse by lying down, deep inspiration, cough, and relieved by sitting up or leaning forward, although other types of chest pain may occur) • Pericarditis rub on examination • New ST-elevation or PR-depression on ECG • New or worsening pericardial effusion on echocardiogram or CMR OR • Autopsy cases may be classified as pericarditis based on meeting histopathologic criteria of the pericardium

[a] Clinical symptoms are for adolescents and adults. Infants and children younger than 12 years night instead have greater than or equal to 2 of the following symptoms: irritability, vomiting, poor feeding, tachypnea, and lethargy. Individuals who lack the listed symptoms but who meet other criteria may be classified as subclinical myocarditis (probable or confirmed).
[b] Using the Lake Lousie criteria.
[c] To meet the ECG or rhythm monitoring criterion, a probable case must include at least one of the following: (1) ST-segment or T-wave abnormailities; (2) paroxysmal or sustained atrail, superventricular, or ventricular arrhythmias; or (3) AV nodal conduction delays or intraventricular conduction defects.
Adapted from Gargano JW, Wallace M, Hadler SC, et al. Use of mRNA COVID-19 Vaccine After Reports of Myocarditis Among Vaccine Recipients: Update from the Advisory Committee on Immunization Practices — United States, June 2021. MMWR Morb Mortal Wkly Rep 2021;70:977–982; *and from* Bozkurt B., Kamat I. and Hotez P.J., Myocarditis with COVID-19 mRNA vaccines, *Circulation*, **144** (6), 2021, 471–484.

compared with 46 for men aged 12 to 15 years and 70 for men aged 16 to 17 years after the second dose. For women, rates were 2, 4, and 8 in the same age ranges, respectively.[18] The vaccine formulation of the Pfizer mRNA vaccine for ages 5 to 11 years of age is one-third the dose of the formulation for those aged 12 years and older, which raises the possibility of a weight-based dose–response relationship in younger adolescents who have lower body weight compared with adults.

Risk with different vaccinations

Among mRNA-based COVID-19 vaccines, the risk of myocarditis is higher following the Moderna vaccine compared with the Pfizer-BioNTech COVID-19 vaccine, although absolute cases numbers vary depending on local availability of each vaccine.[7,19] A study of more than 2.5 million people who received the Pfizer-BioNTech COVID-19 vaccine demonstrated an estimated incidence of myocarditis of 2.1 cases per 100,000 persons,[13] whereas a study of nearly 500,000 people vaccinated with the Moderna vaccine demonstrated an incidence of 4.2 cases per 100,000 persons.[7] A large population-based study in Denmark found that the rates of myocarditis among individuals aged 12 to 39 years were 1.6 per 100,000 individuals for Pfizer-BioNTech and 5.7 per 100,000 individuals for Moderna.[7]

Myocarditis is much more common following the second dose compared with the first but has also been reported following the first dose particularly in those with a prior history of COVID-19 infection.[4] There are limited data on the risk of myocarditis following third and subsequent booster doses.[20,21] However, the risk after the third dose seems to be lower than following the second dose.[14,22] History of prior exposure is likely relevant as well as shorter interval between doses.[23] There are a few case reports of recurrent myocarditis following administration of mRNA-based COVID-19 vaccines.[24,25] However, the risk of recurrence of myocarditis following receipt of additional doses of mRNA COVID-19 vaccines in individuals with a history of confirmed myocarditis is currently unknown.[26] One preprint article suggests that the risk of myocarditis among individuals who received the Moderna vaccine for the second dose was higher for those who had a heterologous as opposed to homologous vaccine schedule (ie, higher in those who had received a COVID-19 vaccine other than the Moderna vaccine for their first dose).[23]

Risk Relative to COVID-19 Infection

Infection with SARS-CoV-2 can also result in myocardial inflammation, which is associated with adverse outcomes in hospitalized patients, and should be balanced against the risk of vaccine-related complications.[27] Overall, the rates of myocarditis following SARS-CoV-2 infection are much higher than after vaccination.[17] Data from the largest integrated health care organization in Israel indicate that SARS-CoV-2 infection is associated with an excess risk of myocarditis when compared with age- and risk-matched controls (risk ratio 18.3 and risk difference 11.0 events per 100,000 persons) that is much higher than the excess risk of myocarditis following administration of Pfizer-BioNTech COVID-19 vaccine (risk ratio 3.2 and risk difference 2.7 events per 100,000 persons).[28] Similarly, higher risk of myocarditis after SARS-CoV-2 infection compared with COVID-19 vaccination was recently demonstrated in a study in England that evaluated more than 38 million individuals aged 16 years and older who had received at least one dose of a COVID-19 vaccine.[9] The extent of abnormalities on cardiac MRI (CMR) is also less severe in myocarditis following COVID-19 vaccination compared with myocarditis following SARS-CoV-2 infection.[29]

Clinical Presentation

Symptoms
The clinical presentation of myocarditis following COVID-19 vaccination is similar to that of myocarditis due to other causes (see **Table 1**). Chest pain is the most frequently reported presenting symptom.[19,30–32] However, as with myocarditis from other causes, myocarditis following COVID-19 vaccination can present with variable symptoms ranging from subclinical presentations to acute arrythmia, heart failure, or rarely cardiogenic shock.[3,13,19]

Timing after vaccination
Most patients with myocarditis following COVID-19 vaccination demonstrate symptom onset within the first week after vaccination, with the vast majority presenting within the first 4 days[19,33–35]; this is similar to myocarditis following non-COVID vaccination where symptom onset is usually less than 2 weeks after vaccine administration.[11,12]

Histopathology and Pathophysiology

Histopathology
Endomyocardial biopsy is not frequently performed in the setting of acute myocarditis but is indicated in patients with suspected myocarditis when diagnostic confirmation will alter therapy, in cases of hemodynamic instability or with clinical deterioration despite supportive care.[36] A negative endomyocardial biopsy does not exclude the diagnosis of myocarditis, given sampling imprecision associated with spatial heterogeneity (patchiness) of the disease.[3,36–38] However, it should also be noted that cardiac dysfunction mimicking myocarditis may result from a systemic increase in cytokine production, which does not have a histological correlate.[37,39–41]

There are very few reports of histologically documented myocarditis following COVID-19 vaccination in the literature to date. Lymphocytic myocarditis is the predominant pattern observed in biopsied and autopsied hearts and occurs most frequently in adolescents and young adult men who present with mild, self-limited disease.[3,41–43] In rare instances it may manifest as a fulminant, potentially fatal disease with no sex predilection.[44–46] Depending on the timing of histologic assessment, a pattern of healing myocarditis may be present. Ameratunga and colleagues report a 57-year-old woman who died of fulminant necrotizing eosinophilic myocarditis 3 days after a first dose of the Pfizer-BioNTech COVID-19 vaccine.[47] Interestingly, myocarditis following other viral vaccines, such as smallpox, measles-mumps-rubella, varicella, oral polio, yellow fever, influenza, hepatitis A and B, and human papillomavirus, is usually of the eosinophilic pattern, albeit not typically necrotizing.[3,39,41] Different histologic patterns of myocarditis are summarized in **Fig. 1**.

Potential mechanisms of myocarditis following vaccination
Several possible mechanisms for mRNA-related myocarditis have emerged (**Fig. 2**).[3,33,41,48] Most of

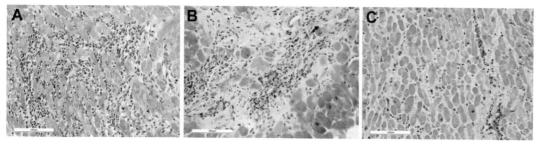

Fig. 1. Examples of different histologic patterns of vaccine-associated myocarditis. (*A*) Lymphocytic myocarditis, the most common pattern reported in COVID-19 vaccination–associated myocarditis, is characterized by a dense mononuclear infiltrate and associated myocyte damage. (*B*) Healing myocarditis is more typically characterized by a loose and more mixed inflammatory infiltrate and with underlying damage already entering stages of repair (matrix formation). (*C*) Eosinophilic myocarditis, the pattern typically associated with other vaccinations, is characterized by a patchy infiltrate of eosinophils with relatively little cardiomyocyte damage. All images are hematoxylin and eosin (H&E)-stained slides, digital image capture (Leica DM2500 microscope, 200x original magnification with 10x Plan ocular and 20x FluorTar objective, OMAX 18MP camera, Toupview software, post-processing in GNU Image Manipulator Program 2.0); scale bar as indicated (100 μm).

them focus on humoral (antibody-mediated) immunity, which is in keeping with the increased prevalence of myocarditis following the second dose of COVID-19 vaccines. One hypothesis involves molecular mimicry between the mRNA vaccine–encoded SARS-CoV2 spike glycoprotein and self-antigens in individuals with preexisting immune dysregulation, leading to polyclonal B-cell expansion, immune complex formation, and inflammation. Alternate explanations involve binding of mRNA vaccine–encoded viral spike glycoprotein to the surface of cardiomyocytes via angiotensin-converting enzyme 2 (ACE2) receptors or deposited immune complexes, thus directly acting as an antigenic trigger for inflammation. Yet another hypothesis involves production of antibodies targeting the anti-spike protein antibodies (ie, antiantibodies), which

mimic the spike protein, bind cardiac ACE2 receptors, form immune complexes, and activate the classic complement pathway. Humoral mechanisms, however, fail to explain the case of a 40-year-old man with biopsy-proven lymphocytic myocarditis in the absence of serum SARS-CoV2 neutralizing antibodies 6 days after receiving a first dose of the Pfizer-BioNTech mRNA COVID-19 vaccine.[42] Consequently, a subset of postvaccine myocarditis might be caused by an innate inflammatory response to the mRNA-encoded viral spike glycoprotein. Testosterone could play a role in the inhibition of antiinflammatory cells or the stimulation of immune responses mediated by Th1 lymphocytes.[49]

Two additional mechanisms not described in the literature still warrant consideration. Theoretically,

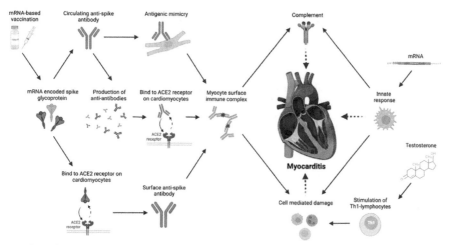

Fig. 2. Potential mechanisms of myocarditis following COVID-19 mRNA vaccination. Overview of the potential mechanisms of myocarditis related to mRNA-based COVID-19 vaccination. ACE, angiotensin-converting enzyme; Th1, helper T cell. Created with BioRender.com.

Table 2
Diagnostic test findings in acute myocarditis

Test	Typical Findings	Strengths	Limitations
Cardiac Imaging			
CMR	• Typically evaluated using the revised Lake Louise criteria • T2-based criteria for myocardial edema include high native T2 and regional T2 hyperintensity • T1-based criteria for myocardial injury include high native T1, high ECV, and nonischemic pattern LGE • +/− Impaired regional and global ventricular function • +/− Pericardial effusion, edema, and enhancement	• High diagnostic sensitivity and specificity for acute myocarditis • Useful in ruling out other potential diagnoses, such as stress-induced cardiomyopathy • Useful in risk stratification • Useful to demonstrate resolution of edema at follow-up	• Limited availability • Relatively long examination time
Echocardiography	• Impaired regional and global ventricular function • Pericardial effusion • +/− Focal echogenicity • +/− Left ventricular dilatation • +/− Impaired strain	• Widely available • Relatively low cost • Relatively short examination time	• Low sensitivity and specificity for myocarditis • Operator dependent
Cardiac CT	• Pericardial effusion or thickening • +/− Myocardial wall thickening • Late iodine enhancement	• Useful in ruling out other potential diagnoses that might present similarly, such as stress-induced cardiomyopathy	• Exposure to ionizing radiation • Low specificity for acute myocarditis
Cardiac PET	• Focal FDG uptake indicates myocardial inflammation	• Metabolic information • Potentially useful in monitoring treatment response	• Limited availability • Exposure to ionizing radiation
Chest radiography	• Possible cardiomegaly • Pericardial effusion • Pulmonary edema in the setting of heart failure	• Widely available • Low cost • Very short examination time • Useful in ruling out other causes of symptoms	• Findings are not specific for myocarditis
Other Investigations			
Troponin	• Elevated values indicate myocyte injury	• Elevated in almost all patients with acute myocarditis • Widely available	• Requires blood draw • Not specific for acute myocarditis

(continued on next page)

Table 2
(continued)

Test	Typical Findings	Strengths	Limitations
BNP	• Elevated values are associated with heart failure	• Widely available	• Requires blood draw • Not specific for acute myocarditis
ECG	• ST-segment and T-wave abnormalities	• Widely available • Relatively quick • Useful in ruling out other potential diagnoses that might present similarly	• Not specific for acute myocarditis
Endomyocardial biopsy	• Inflammatory infiltrates within the myocardium associated with myocyte damage/necrosis of nonischemic origin • Newer criteria may use immunohistochemical techniques	• Reference standard for definitive diagnosis of myocarditis • High specificity	• Invasive with risk of complications • Low sensitivity for acute myocarditis due to sampling error and patchy disease

Abbreviations: BNP, brain natriuretic peptide; CMR, cardiac magnetic resonance; CT, computed tomography; ECG, echocardiography; ECV, extracellular volume; FDG, fluorodeoxyglucose; LGE, late gadolinium enhancement; PET, positron emission tomography.

vaccine mRNA can enter circulation, rather than being directly expressed at the injection site, and could become expressed in cardiomyocytes and thus trigger direct cell-mediated responses against spike protein.[50] In addition, despite chemical modifications and liposome delivery to prevent such, exogenous RNA can trigger the innate immune response, causing activation of the cellular inflammasome and acting as an adjuvant to antigen-mediated responses.[51]

Role of Cardiac Imaging

A summary of diagnostic test findings in acute myocarditis is provided in **Table 2**. Cardiac imaging plays an important role in establishing a diagnosis of myocarditis and pericarditis, excluding other potential causes of symptoms, and risk-stratifying patients.

Echocardiography

Transthoracic echocardiography is often the first cardiac imaging modality performed in the setting of suspected myocarditis, allowing for assessment of cardiac size and function and associated findings including the presence of a pericardial effusion. Although most findings in the setting of myocarditis are not specific, focal echogenicity, particularly in the lateral and inferior wall, and the presence of pericardial effusions have been shown to be sensitive for acute myopericarditis in young adults.[52] Speckle tracking–based myocardial strain is also a potentially sensitive method to identify acute myocarditis with echocardiography.[53] Impaired ventricular function is a predictor of poor outcomes, and echocardiography is also useful in follow-up to ensure recovery of function[54]

Cardiac computed tomography

Cardiac computed tomography (CT) is infrequently used in the evaluation of suspected myocarditis but can be helpful in excluding other potential causes of acute chest pain, including obstructive coronary artery disease. In the setting of an inability to perform CMR, late iodine enhancement on CT could be considered, given high sensitivity and positive predictive value for acute myocarditis.[55]

Cardiac positron emission tomography

Cardiac fluorodeoxyglucose PET (FDG-PET) is useful in the evaluation of cardiac inflammation and is most often used clinically in the setting of cardiac sarcoidosis.[56] However, focal cardiac FDG uptake on PET has also been described in the setting of myocardial inflammation due to other causes including COVID-19 infection.[57] Combined cardiac PET/MR adds complementary information and increases the sensitivity for mild or borderline myocarditis compared with CMR, although not widely available.[57–60]

Cardiac magnetic resonance imaging

CMR is the most important imaging modality for diagnosis of acute myocarditis. The Lake Louise criteria are most commonly used for evaluation of suspected myocarditis on CMR. These criteria were initially established in 2009 and were revised in 2018 to incorporate parametric mapping.[61] The revised criteria indicate a high likelihood of nonischemic myocardial inflammation when at least one of each of the T1- and T2-based criteria are met. T1-based criteria include increased native T1, increased extracellular volume (ECV), or presence of nonischemic pattern late gadolinium enhancement (LGE). T2-based criteria include increased native T2, regional T2 hyperintensity, or increased myocardial T2 signal intensity ratio compared with skeletal muscle on T2-weighted imaging. Regional and global left ventricular dysfunction and findings associated with pericarditis (including presence of a pericardial effusion and pericardial enhancement) are supportive criteria but are not required.

Although the presence of both T1- and T2-based criteria is associated with the highest specificity for active myocardial inflammation, the presence of only one criterion could still be consistent with a diagnosis of myocarditis, particularly if imaging was delayed after symptom onset or performed after immunosuppressive treatment is started (in which case edema might no longer be detectable).[4] Given the importance of establishing a diagnosis of myocarditis, CMR should ideally be performed as soon as possible after the onset of symptoms; this may be particularly relevant in the setting of myocarditis following COVID-19 vaccination, given reports of very rapid resolution of symptoms and the potential implications of a diagnosis on recommendations for future vaccination.[4]

In acute myocarditis in general, LGE most commonly occurs in a subepicardial pattern and is often located at the basal inferior lateral wall. Mid-wall and septal patterns of LGE are less common but are associated with a worse prognosis.[62] Myocardial edema is usually focal; however, diffuse changes have also been described.[63] In the acute setting, LGE co-localizing with edema is often associated with functional recovery, as edema improves over time.[64] However, isolated LGE without edema often reflects fibrosis, which is a risk marker for major cardiac events including sudden cardiac death and heart failure.[64] Native T1, T2, and ECV allow for quantification of myocardial tissue changes and are all elevated in the setting of myocardial edema. On the other hand, elevation of T1 and ECV in the setting of normal T2 values suggests healed myocarditis with fibrosis but no active edema.[4]

The pattern of CMR findings in myocarditis following COVID-19 vaccination is similar to myocarditis due to other causes, although the extent and severity of abnormalities tends to be milder.[4] Typical findings in the acute phase include subepicardial LGE and co-localizing edema at the basal to mid-inferolateral wall, **Fig. 3**. Compared with other causes of myocarditis, patients with vaccine-associated myocarditis have higher left ventricular ejection fraction, less extensive LGE, and less frequent involvement of the septum.[29]

Follow-up CMR is often performed 3 to 6 months after acute myocarditis to evaluate for recovery of left ventricular function, resolution of edema, and any residual scarring, although there are no established guidelines defining the optimal timing of follow-up imaging.[65] There are limited follow-up CMR data in myocarditis following vaccination.[66–69] In a case series of 13 adults with acute myocarditis following COVID-19 vaccination, intermediate-term follow-up CMR at a median of 5 months demonstrated resolution of myocardial edema, normalization of left ventricular function, and interval decrease in LGE extent (**Fig. 4**).[66] However, minimal residual LGE without edema was present in 8 out of 13 patients at follow-up, likely reflecting myocardial fibrosis. Similarly, in a case series of 16 pediatric patients with myocarditis following COVID-19 vaccination, follow-up CMR at a median of 3 months demonstrated normalization of LVEF and interval decrease in LGE extent.[67] However, minimal LGE persisted in 11 out of 16 and global longitudinal strain remained impaired in 12 out of 16. Longer-term follow-up in larger cohorts of patients is needed to understand the sequelae of myocarditis following vaccination and the ability of imaging abnormalities to identify patients who are at risk of adverse cardiac events.

Other Investigations

Other diagnostic investigations used frequently in the setting of myocarditis and pericarditis include electrocardiography (ECG) and assessment of cardiac blood biomarkers. ECG findings in myocarditis are nonspecific but can include ST-segment elevation, T-wave inversions, and ectopic beats.[31,34,70] Although these findings have low sensitivity for myocarditis, ECG is frequently used in patients with suspected myocarditis to evaluate for alternative causes of cardiac symptoms.[70] In the setting of pericarditis, typical ECG changes include concave upward ST-segment elevation, upright T waves in the leads with ST-segment elevation, and PR depression. ECG findings in the setting of myocarditis and pericarditis following COVID-19 vaccination are similar to other causes.[19,70]

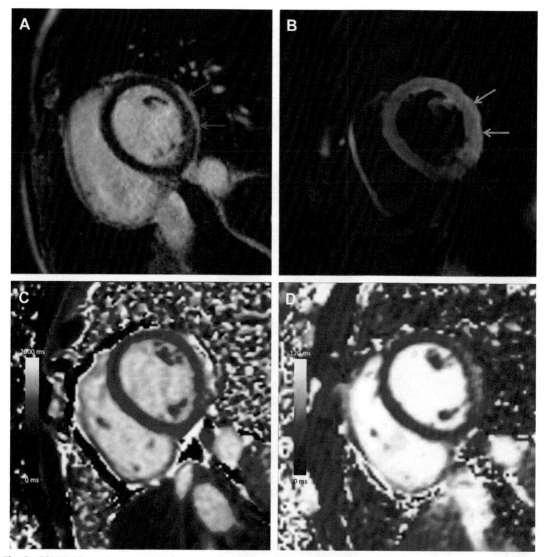

Fig. 3. COVID-19 vaccine–associated myocarditis. Short-axis 1.5 T MRI images of a young adult man with myocarditis following mRNA COVID-19 vaccine administration demonstrating (*A*) subepicardial late gadolinium enhancement (LGE) at the basal to mid-inferior lateral wall (*red arrows*), with corresponding (*B*) hyperintensity on T2-weighted imaging (*orange arrows*), (*C*) abnormal high native T1 (1274 ms, maximum region of interest), and (*D*) abnormal high native T2 (65 ms, maximum region of interest).

Although not specific to myocarditis, elevated troponin levels, indicating myocyte injury, are almost always present in the setting of acute myocarditis.[3,19,30,71] The degree of troponin elevation varies and depends the severity of myocardial injury and timing of evaluation in relation to symptom onset. Elevated brain natriuretic peptide (BNP) levels indicate increased ventricular stretch and are elevated in the setting of heart failure. BNP is often assessed in patients with suspected myocarditis when heart failure symptoms are present. However, elevations of BNP are not included in the CDC working case definitions of probable or confirmed acute myocarditis, and values are not consistently evaluated or reported. Other testing, such as acute and convalescent viral testing (eg, SARS-CoV-2, coxsackievirus, and so forth), should be considered when clinically appropriate to exclude other potential causes of myocarditis.

Management
Currently, there are no specific management recommendations for myocarditis following COVID-19 vaccination. Care is largely supportive following guidelines for myocarditis due to other causes.[39] Treatment is typically focused on addressing potential sequelae such as heart failure or arrhythmia as per guideline-directed medical therapy. For

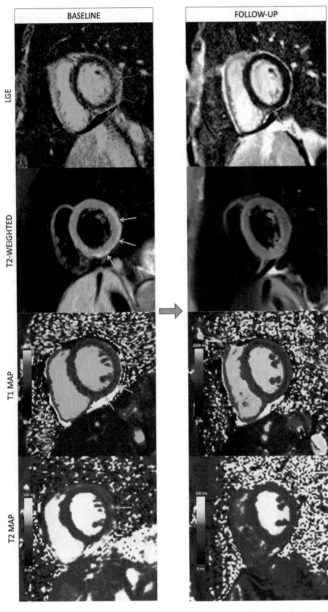

Fig. 4. Baseline and follow-up CMR in COVID-19 vaccine–associated myocarditis. Short-axis cardiac MRI images in a young adult man with myocarditis following the second dose of mRNA-1273. Baseline MRI at 1.5 T demonstrates subepicardial late gadolinium enhancement (LGE) at the basal inferior and inferolateral wall (*red arrows*) with corresponding high T2 signal in keeping with edema (*yellow arrows*), high regional native T1 (*green arrows*), and high regional T2 (*blue arrows*). Follow-up cardiac MRI performed 4 months later at 3 T demonstrates interval decrease in LGE extent (*orange arrow*) with resolution of edema and normalization of T1 and T2 values.

patients with very mild symptoms with rapid improvement, therapy can often be deferred.

Individuals are typically safe to return to their normal daily activities after their symptoms improve. However, the optimal duration of exercise restriction is unknown. The American Heart Association and American College of Cardiology Foundation have recommended 3 to 6 months of restriction from competitive sports following myocarditis. Repeat evaluation of serum biomarkers, 24-hour Holter monitor, and echocardiography is recommended before return to exercise in order to ensure normal ventricular function, resolution of active inflammation, and absence of arrhythmias.[72]

Although there is no clear evidence on risk associated with subsequent vaccination, current guidelines suggest that further doses of mRNA COVID-19 vaccines should be deferred among individuals who experienced myocarditis within 6 weeks of receiving a previous dose of an mRNA COVID-19 vaccine.[26]

Clinical Course and Adverse Outcomes

Myocarditis following COVID-19 vaccination is typically associated with a transient, mild course, with complete resolution of symptoms within 1 to 3 weeks in most of the patients.[3,19,30,34] Patients with more severe disease with ventricular dysfunction might require hospitalization, although most reports indicate that patients who do require hospitalization typically require a short stay of less than 5 days.[19,34] Patients rarely require intensive care unit admission or readmission following hospital discharge.[12]

Although most patients with myocarditis after COVID-19 vaccination have a mild course, there are limited long-term follow-up data, given the relatively recent introduction of these vaccines. Improvement or normalization of ejection fraction and resolution of symptoms in nearly all patients with myocarditis following COVID-19 vaccination has been demonstrated at short-interval follow-up.[12] Limited intermediate term (~5–6 months) follow-up data have demonstrated normalization of troponin levels, no residual cardiac symptoms or functional impairment, and no adverse cardiac events.[66,68] Although these data are reassuring, further studies with long-term clinical and imaging follow-up are needed. Additional study is also needed to determine the risk with subsequent vaccine doses and other potential risk factors including prior history of myocarditis.

SUMMARY

Myocarditis is an established but rare adverse event following administration of mRNA-based COVID-19 vaccines, with highest risk in male adolescents and young adults. Symptoms typically develop within a few days of vaccine administration. Most patients have mild abnormalities on cardiac imaging with rapid clinical improvement with standard treatment, which is reassuring. However, longer term follow-up is needed to determine whether imaging abnormalities persist, to evaluate for adverse outcomes, and to understand the risk associated with subsequent vaccination.

CLINICS CARE POINTS

- Myocarditis following mRNA-based COVID-19 vaccines is rare; however, adolescent and young adult men are at highest risk.
- Chest pain is the most common symptom, with typical onset within a few days of vaccine administration.
- CMR plays an important role in the diagnosis of acute myocarditis following vaccination, with typical findings of subepicardial late gadolinium enhancement and co-localizing edema at the basal inferior lateral wall.

- The disease course of myocarditis following COVID-19 vaccination is typically transient and mild, with resolution of symptoms within 1 to 3 weeks in most patients.
- However, longer term follow-up is needed to determine whether imaging abnormalities persist, to evaluate for adverse outcomes, and to understand the risk associated with subsequent vaccination.

FUNDING

Dr P. Thavendiranathan is supported by a Canada Research Chair. Dr J.A. Udell is supported by a Department of Medicine, University of Toronto Merit Award and receives support from Ontario Ministry of Colleges and Universities Early Researcher Award (ER15-11-037).

DISCLOSURE

Dr K. Hanneman has received speaker's honorarium from Sanofi-Genzyme, Amicus, and Medscape. Dr P. Thavendiranathan has received speaker's honorarium from Amgen, Boehringer Ingelheim-Lilly, and Takeda. Dr J.A. Udell has served as a consultant or speaker for AstraZeneca, Bayer, Boehringer Ingelheim-Lilly, Janssen, Merck, Novartis, and Sanofi and has received research grants from AstraZeneca, Amgen, Bayer, Boehringer Ingelheim-Lilly, and Janssen.

REFERENCES

1. Hanneman K, Iwanochko RM, Thavendiranathan P. Evolution of lymphadenopathy at PET/MRI after COVID-19 vaccination. Radiology 2021;299(3): E282.
2. See I, Su JR, Lale A, et al. US Case reports of cerebral venous sinus thrombosis with thrombocytopenia after Ad26.COV2.S vaccination, March 2 to April 21, 2021. JAMA 2021;325(24):2448–56.
3. Bozkurt B, Kamat I, Hotez PJ. Myocarditis with COVID-19 mRNA vaccines. Circulation 2021; 144(6):471–84.
4. Sanchez Tijmes F, Thavendiranathan P, Udell JA, et al. Cardiac MRI assessment of nonischemic myocardial inflammation: state of the art review and update on myocarditis associated with COVID-19 vaccination. Radiol Cardiothorac Imaging 2021;3(6):e210252.
5. Caforio AL, Pankuweit S, Arbustini E, et al. Current state of knowledge on aetiology, diagnosis, management, and therapy of ˙myocarditis: a position statement of the european society of cardiology

working group on myocardial and pericardial diseases. Eur Heart J 2013;34(33):2636–48, 48a-48d.

6. Su JR, McNeil MM, Welsh KJ, et al. Myopericarditis after vaccination, vaccine adverse event reporting system (VAERS), 1990-2018. Vaccine 2021;39(5):839–45.

7. Husby A, Hansen JV, Fosbol E, et al. SARS-CoV-2 vaccination and myocarditis or myopericarditis: population based cohort study. BMJ 2021;375: e068665.

8. Mevorach D, Anis E, Cedar N, et al. Myocarditis after BNT162b2 mRNA vaccine against covid-19 in Israel. N Engl J Med 2021;385(23):2140–9.

9. Patone M, Mei XW, Handunnetthi L, et al. Risks of myocarditis, pericarditis, and cardiac arrhythmias associated with COVID-19 vaccination or SARS-CoV-2 infection. Nat Med 2021;28(2):410–22.

10. Perez Y, Levy ER, Joshi AY, et al. Myocarditis following COVID-19 mRNA vaccine: a case series and incidence rate determination. Clin Infect Dis 2021;3:ciab926.

11. United States Department of Health and Human Services (DHHS). Public health service (PHS), centers for disease control (CDC)/food and Drug administration (FDA), vaccine adverse event reporting system (VAERS) 1990 - 01/07/2022. CDC WONDER On-line Database [cited 2022 January 16]. Available at: http://wonder.cdc.gov/vaers.

12. Simone A, Herald J, Chen A, et al. Acute myocarditis following COVID-19 mRNA vaccination in adults aged 18 years or older. JAMA Intern Med 2021; 181(12):1668–70.

13. Witberg G, Barda N, Hoss S, et al. Myocarditis after Covid-19 vaccination in a large health care organization. N Engl J Med 2021;385(23):2132–9.

14. Ling RR, Ramanathan K, Tan FL, et al. Myopericarditis following COVID-19 vaccination and non- COVID-19 vaccination: a systematic review and meta-analysis. Lancet Respir Med 2022;11(22):S2213–600, 00059-5.

15. Hajjo R, Sabbah DA, Bardaweel SK, et al. Shedding the light on post-vaccine myocarditis and pericarditis in COVID-19 and non-COVID-19 vaccine recipients. Vaccines 2021;9(10).

16. Oster ME, Shay DK, Su JR, et al. Myocarditis cases reported after mRNA-based COVID-19 vaccination in the US from december 2020 to august 2021. JAMA 2022;327(4):331–40.

17. Gargano JW, Wallace M, Hadler SC, et al. Use of mRNA COVID-19 vaccine after reports of myocarditis among vaccine recipients: update from the advisory committee on immunization practices - United States, june 2021. MMWR Morb Mortal Wkly Rep 2021;70(27):977–82.

18. Su JR. COVID-19 vaccine safety updates: primary series in children and adolescents ages 5–11 and 12–15 years, and booster doses in adolescents ages 16–24 years 2022 [cited 2022 January 20].

Available at: https://www.cdc.gov/vaccines/acip/meetings/downloads/slides-2022-01-05/02-covid-su-508.pdf.

19. Montgomery J, Ryan M, Engler R, et al. Myocarditis following immunization with mRNA COVID-19 Vaccines in members of the US military. JAMA Cardiol 2021;6(10):1202–6.

20. Aviram G, Viskin D, Topilsky Y, et al. Myocarditis associated with COVID-19 booster vaccination. Circ Cardiovasc Imaging 2022;15(2):e013771.

21. Sanchez Tijmes F, Zamorano A, Thavendiranathan P, et al. Imaging of myocarditis following mRNA COVID-19 booster vaccination. Radiol Cardiothorac Imaging 2022;4(2):e220019.

22. Friedensohn L, Levin D, Fadlon-Derai M, et al. Myocarditis following a third BNT162b2 vaccination dose in military recruits in Israel. JAMA 2022;17: e224425.

23. Buchan SA, Seo CY, Johnson C, et al. Epidemiology of myocarditis and pericarditis following mRNA vaccines in Ontario, Canada: by vaccine product, schedule and interval. medRxiv 2021;2021.

24. Minocha PK, Better D, Singh RK, et al. Recurrence of acute myocarditis temporally associated with receipt of the mRNA coronavirus disease 2019 (COVID-19) vaccine in a male adolescent. J Pediatr 2021;238:321–3.

25. Umei TC, Kishino Y, Shiraishi Y, et al. Recurrence of myopericarditis following mRNA COVID-19 vaccination in a male adolescent. CJC Open 2022;4(3):350–2.

26. Summary of NACI advice on vaccination with COVID-19. vaccines following myocarditis (with or without pericarditis) [cited 2022 January 28]. Available at: https://www.canada.ca/en/public-health/services/immunization/national-advisory-committee-on-immunization-naci/summary-advice-vaccination-covid-19-vaccines-following-myocarditis-with-without-pericarditis.html.

27. Guo T, Fan Y, Chen M, et al. Cardiovascular implications of fatal outcomes of patients with coronavirus disease 2019 (COVID-19). JAMA Cardiol 2020; 5(7):811–8.

28. Barda N, Dagan N, Ben-Shlomo Y, et al. Safety of the BNT162b2 mRNA Covid-19 vaccine in a nationwide setting. N Engl J Med 2021;385(12):1078–90.

29. Fronza MT, Thavendiranathan P, Chan V, et al. Myocardial injury pattern by MRI in COVID-19 vaccine associated myocarditis. Radiology 2022;15:212559.

30. Engler RJ, Nelson MR, Collins LC Jr, et al. A prospective study of the incidence of myocarditis/pericarditis and new onset cardiac symptoms following smallpox and influenza vaccination. PLoS One 2015;10(3):e0118283.

31. Halsell JS, Riddle JR, Atwood JE, et al. Myopericarditis following smallpox vaccination among vaccinia-naive US military personnel. JAMA 2003;289(24): 3283–9.

32. Mei R, Raschi E, Forcesi E, et al. Myocarditis and pericarditis after immunization: gaining insights through the vaccine adverse event reporting system. Int J Cardiol 2018;273:183–6.

33. Heymans S, Cooper LT. Myocarditis after COVID-19 mRNA vaccination: clinical observations and potential mechanisms. Nat Rev Cardiol 2022;19:75077.

34. Das BB, Moskowitz WB, Taylor MB, et al. Myocarditis and pericarditis following mRNA COVID-19 vaccination: what do we know so far? Children (Basel) 2021; 8(7):607.

35. Matta A, Kunadharaju R, Osman M, et al. Clinical presentation and outcomes of myocarditis post mRNA vaccination: a meta-analysis and systematic review. Cureus 2021;13(11):e19240.

36. Leone O, Veinot JP, Angelini A, et al. 2011 Consensus statement on endomyocardial biopsy from the association for european cardiovascular pathology and the society for cardiovascular pathology. Cardiovasc Pathol 2012;21(4):245–74.

37. Baughman KL. Diagnosis of myocarditis: death of Dallas criteria. Circulation 2006;113(4):593–5.

38. Chow LH, Radio SJ, Sears TD, et al. Insensitivity of right ventricular endomyocardial biopsy in the diagnosis of myocarditis. J Am Coll Cardiol 1989;14(4): 915–20.

39. Luk A, Clarke B, Dahdah N, et al. Myocarditis and pericarditis after COVID-19 mRNA vaccination: practical considerations for care providers. Can J Cardiol 2021;37(10):1629–34.

40. Rali AS, Ranka S, Shah Z, et al. Mechanisms of myocardial injury in coronavirus disease 2019. Card Fail Rev 2020;6:e15.

41. Switzer C, Loeb M. Evaluating the relationship between myocarditis and mRNA vaccination. Expert Rev Vaccin 2022;21(1):83–9.

42. Ehrlich P, Klingel K, Ohlmann-Knafo S, et al. Biopsy-proven lymphocytic myocarditis following first mRNA COVID-19 vaccination in a 40-year-old male: case report. Clin Res Cardiol 2021;110(11): 1855–9.

43. Jain SS, Steele JM, Fonseca B, et al. COVID-19 vaccination-associated myocarditis in adolescents. Pediatrics 2021;148(5).

44. Abbate A, Gavin J, Madanchi N, et al. Fulminant myocarditis and systemic hyperinflammation temporally associated with BNT162b2 mRNA COVID-19 vaccination in two patients. Int J Cardiol 2021;340: 119–21.

45. Lim Y, Kim MC, Kim KH, et al. Case report: acute fulminant myocarditis and cardiogenic shock after messenger RNA coronavirus disease 2019 vaccination requiring extracorporeal cardiopulmonary resuscitation. Front Cardiovasc Med 2021;8:758996.

46. Verma AK, Lavine KJ, Lin CY. Myocarditis after covid-19 mRNA vaccination. N Engl J Med 2021; 385(14):1332–4.

47. Ameratunga R, Woon ST, Sheppard MN, et al. First identified case of fatal fulminant necrotizing eosinophilic myocarditis following the initial dose of the pfizer-biontech mRNA COVID-19 vaccine (BNT162b2, Comirnaty): an extremely rare idiosyncratic hypersensitivity reaction. J Clin Immunol 2022;3:1–7.

48. Kadkhoda K. Post RNA-based COVID vaccines myocarditis: proposed mechanisms. Vaccine 2022; 40(3):406–7.

49. Lazaros G, Klein AL, Hatziantoniou S, et al. The novel platform of mRNA COVID-19 vaccines and myocarditis: clues into the potential underlying mechanism. Vaccine 2021;39(35):4925–7.

50. Rijkers GT, Weterings N, Obregon-Henao A, et al. Antigen presentation of mRNA-based and virus-vectored SARS-CoV-2 vaccines. Vaccines (Basel) 2021;9(8).

51. Milano G, Gal J, Creisson A, et al. Myocarditis and COVID-19 mRNA vaccines: a mechanistic hypothesis involving dsRNA. Future Virol 2022;17(3): 191–6.

52. Saricam E, Saglam Y, Hazirolan T. Clinical evaluation of myocardial involvement in acute myopericarditis in young adults. BMC Cardiovasc Disord 2017; 17(1):129.

53. Hsiao JF, Koshino Y, Bonnichsen CR, et al. Speckle tracking echocardiography in acute myocarditis. Int J Cardiovasc Imaging 2013; 29(2):275–84.

54. van den Heuvel FMA, Vos JL, van Bakel B, et al. Comparison between myocardial function assessed by echocardiography during hospitalization for COVID-19 and at 4 months follow-up. Int J Cardiovasc Imaging 2021;37(12):3459–67.

55. Bouleti C, Baudry G, Iung B, et al. Usefulness of late iodine enhancement on spectral CT in acute myocarditis. JACC Cardiovasc Imaging 2017; 10(7):826–7.

56. Genovesi D, Bauckneht M, Altini C, et al. The role of positron emission tomography in the assessment of cardiac sarcoidosis. Br J Radiol 2019;92(1100): 20190247.

57. Hanneman K, Houbois C, Schoffel A, et al. Combined cardiac fluorodeoxyglucose-positron emission tomography/magnetic resonance imaging assessment of myocardial injury in patients who recently recovered from COVID-19. JAMA Cardiol 2022;7(3):298–308, 1.

58. Chen W, Jeudy J. Assessment of myocarditis: cardiac MR, PET/CT, or PET/MR? Curr Cardiol Rep 2019;21(8):76.

59. Cheung E, Ahmad S, Aitken M, et al. Combined simultaneous FDG-PET/MRI with T1 and T2 mapping as an imaging biomarker for the diagnosis and prognosis of suspected cardiac sarcoidosis. Eur J Hybrid Imaging 2021;5(1):24.

60. Hanneman K, Kadoch M, Guo HH, et al. Initial experience with simultaneous 18F-FDG PET/MRI in the evaluation of cardiac sarcoidosis and myocarditis. Clin Nucl Med 2017;42(7):e328–34.

61. Ferreira VM, Schulz-Menger J, Holmvang G, et al. Cardiovascular magnetic resonance in nonischemic myocardial inflammation: expert recommendations. J Am Coll Cardiol 2018;72(24):3158–76.

62. Grani C, Eichhorn C, Biere L, et al. Prognostic value of cardiac magnetic resonance tissue characterization in risk stratifying patients with suspected myocarditis. J Am Coll Cardiol 2017;70(16):1964–76.

63. Luetkens JA, Isaak A, Zimmer S, et al. Diffuse myocardial inflammation in COVID-19 associated myocarditis detected by multiparametric cardiac magnetic resonance imaging. Circ Cardiovasc Imaging 2020;13(5):e010897.

64. Aquaro GD, Ghebru Habtemicael Y, Camastra G, et al. Prognostic value of repeating cardiac magnetic resonance in patients with acute myocarditis. J Am Coll Cardiol 2019;74(20):2439–48.

65. Tschope C, Ammirati E, Bozkurt B, et al. Myocarditis and inflammatory cardiomyopathy: current evidence and future directions. Nat Rev Cardiol 2021;18(3):169–93.

66. Fronza M, Thavendiranathan P, Karur GR, et al. Cardiac MRI and clinical follow-up in COVID-19 vaccine associated myocarditis. Radiology 2022;May 3:220802. https://doi.org/10.1148/radiol.220802.

67. Schauer J, Buddhe S, Gulhane A, et al. Persistent cardiac MRI findings in a cohort of adolescents with post COVID-19 mRNA vaccine myopericarditis. J Pediatr 2022;26(22):S0022-3476, 00282-7.

68. Rosner CM, Atkins M, Saeed IM, et al. Patients with myocarditis associated with COVID-19 vaccination. J Am Coll Cardiol 2022;79(13):1317–9.

69. Cavalcante JL, Shaw KE, Gossl M. Cardiac magnetic resonance imaging midterm follow up of covid-19 vaccine–associated myocarditis. JACC Cardiovasc Imaging 2022;16:2022.

70. Kindermann I, Barth C, Mahfoud F, et al. Update on myocarditis. J Am Coll Cardiol 2012;59(9):779–92.

71. Shaw KE, Cavalcante JL, Han BK, et al. Possible association between COVID-19 vaccine and myocarditis: clinical and CMR findings. JACC Cardiovasc Imaging 2021;14(9):1856–61.

72. Maron BJ, Udelson JE, Bonow RO, et al. Eligibility and disqualification recommendations for competitive athletes with cardiovascular abnormalities: task force 3: hypertrophic cardiomyopathy, arrhythmogenic right ventricular cardiomyopathy and other cardiomyopathies, and myocarditis: a scientific statement from the american heart association and american college of cardiology. Circulation 2015;132(22):e273–80.

Cardiovascular Health Care Implications of the COVID-19 pandemic

Zahra Raisi-Estabragh, MD, PhD[a,b], Mamas A. Mamas, MD, DPhil[c,d,e],*

KEYWORDS

- COVID-19 • Cardiovascular disease • Health care provision • Health inequalities
- Population health

KEY POINTS

- There are wide reports of excess cardiovascular mortality particularly during the early phases of the pandemic, largely attributed to primary cardiovascular causes, with notable translocation of deaths from hospitals to the community.
- There has been a significant decline in hospitalizations for acute cardiovascular conditions and related procedures such as percutaneous coronary interventions for acute myocardial infarction and mechanical thrombectomy for strokes.
- There are backlogs in elective cardiovascular procedures, such as aortic valve interventions; delays in such time-sensitive treatments are likely to have a significant adverse prognostic impact.
- There is evidence of substantial treatment deficits in primary and secondary cardiovascular prevention, which, if not addressed, may have a longstanding population-level impact on cardiovascular health.
- The pandemic has highlighted the significant adverse public health impact of health care inequalities, the reduction of which requires concerted efforts in multiple areas of health and social care and cohesive action from policy makers and health care professionals.

INTRODUCTION

The coronavirus disease 2019 (COVID-19) pandemic has placed immense pressure on health care services, necessitating reorganization and reprioritization of resources and changes in models of health care delivery. Large number of COVID-19 inpatient admissions has required restructuring of hospital services and redeployment of staff for the provision of acute clinical care. Furthermore, many governments have postponed nonurgent elective work, due to both staff and infrastructure limitations, as well as concerns around the exposure of potentially vulnerable patients to infection. These service pressures have been further compounded by staff shortages related to COVID-19 infection or contact exposure requiring isolation.

There have also been changes in the public's pattern of health care utilization, owing, in part, to altered risk perceptions and health-seeking behaviors.[1] Such behavioral changes have perhaps been influenced by national "lockdowns" or "stay at home" public health recommendations. Thus, delayed service provision due to resource-

This article originally appeared in Cardiology Clinics, Volume 40, Issue 3, August 2022.
a William Harvey Research Institute, NIHR Barts Biomedical Research Centre, Queen Mary University, London EC1M 6BQ, United Kingdom; b Barts Heart Centre, St Bartholomew's Hospital, Barts Health NHS Trust, West Smithfield, London EC1A 7BE, United Kingdom; c Keele Cardiovascular Research Group, Keele University, Keele ST5 5BG, United Kingdom; d Department of Cardiology, Thomas Jefferson University, Philadelphia, PA 19107, USA; e Institute of Population Health, University of Manchester, Manchester M13 9PT, United kingdom
* Corresponding author. Keele Cardiovascular Research Group, Centre for Prognosis Research, Keele University, Stoke-on-Trent, Keele ST5 5BG, United Kingdom.
E-mail address: mamasmamas1@yahoo.co.uk

Heart Failure Clin 19 (2023) 265–272
https://doi.org/10.1016/j.hfc.2022.08.010
1551-7136/23/© 2022 Elsevier Inc. All rights reserved.

constrained health care delivery systems has been augmented by patients' hesitance to access health care.

Indeed, growing evidence indicates a significant decline in the use of health care services across multiple key areas. In the UK, emergency department (ED) visits declined by 49% and out-of-hours general practice consultations fell by 11% during the peak pandemic period in 2020 compared with the preceding year.[1] In the US, there was a 42% decline in ED visits.[2] Similar trends were seen across Europe and globally. A study of 27 European nations reported a significant reduction in health care utilization after the first COVID-19 outbreak.[3] While reports from China,[4] Singapore,[5] and Taiwan[6] indicate declines in the utilization of both inpatient and outpatient services.

Available evidence suggests major disruptions to the delivery and utilization of cardiovascular services during the pandemic, with important clinical consequences. Cardiovascular diseases are the most common cause of morbidity and mortality worldwide.[7] Their management requires a combination of preventive medicine, acute care, and chronic disease management. The longer-term impact of service disruptions during the pandemic on population cardiovascular health is likely significant and not yet fully appreciated.

In this narrative review, we examine the implications of the COVID-19 pandemic for cardiovascular health care, including excess cardiovascular mortality, acute and elective cardiovascular care, and disease prevention. Additionally, we consider the long-term public health consequences of disruptions to cardiovascular care across both primary and secondary care settings. Finally, we review health care inequalities and their driving factors, as highlighted by the pandemic, and consider their importance in the context of cardiovascular health care.

ACUTE CARDIOVASCULAR CARE

The COVID-19 pandemic has resulted in excess premature mortality across many countries worldwide.[8,9] Cardiovascular disease and its risk factors have been linked to higher risk of adverse COVID-19 outcomes, including more severe disease manifestations and higher risk of death[10–12] (**Fig. 1**). In a meta-analysis of 51 studies including a total of 48,317 patients, Bae and colleagues[10] identified pre-existing cardiovascular risk factors (hypertension, diabetes) and CVD itself as independent predictors of mortality among patients with COVID-19 across all age groups. A large nationwide study from Korea similarly reports significant associations of diabetes, hypertension, and heart failure

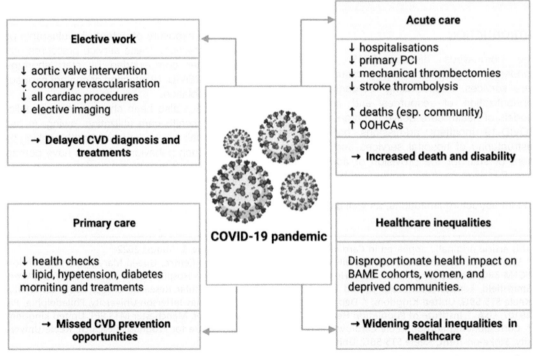

Fig. 1. Central illustration. Impact of COVID-19 on cardiovascular care. BAME, Black Asian and Minority Ethnic; CVD, cardiovascular disease; OOHCA, out-of-hospital cardiac arrest; PCI, percutaneous coronary intervention.

with critical illness among patients hospitalized with COVID-19.[11] Accordingly, Wu and colleagues[13] report an 8% increase in acute cardiovascular deaths in England during the pandemic period. However, the excess cardiovascular deaths are not fully attributed to direct COVID-19 effects. While a proportion of these deaths were related to COVID-19 (5.1%), the most frequent primary causes of death were stroke (35.6%), acute coronary syndrome (ACS, 24.5%), and heart failure (23.4%).[13]

These observations may reflect reduced access to emergency services for these conditions, compounded by the hesitance of patients to seek medical care during the pandemic. In the UK, public health messaging during the early stages of the COVID-19 pandemic centered around the slogan of "stay home, protect the NHS, save lives," with similar variations in other nations, which may have increased the reticence of patients to seek medical attention for acute cardiovascular events. Others have pointed out confusion around hospital protocols as a key reason for delays in seeking treatment for non–COVID-19 illnesses during the pandemic.[14] Wu and colleagues[13] demonstrate a translocation in the place of death, with substantial increases in cardiovascular deaths at home (+35%) and in care homes or hospices (+32%), with more modest increase in hospital deaths. Mafham and colleagues,[15] also report a significant decline in the number of patients hospitalized with ACS per week in England at the end of March 2020 compared with weekly prepandemic averages. Braiteh and colleagues[16] report similar trends from the US with 40.7% reduction in total hospital admission for ACS. There is also evidence that patients who did seek medical help waited significantly longer to do so compared with the prepandemic period. In a study from Switzerland, Nils and colleagues[17] report both a significant decline in the incidence of ACS and prolonged delays from symptom onset to time of first medical contact. Studies from the US and Germany report similar experiences of increased delays in time to presentation for ACS.[18,19] Such treatment delays have important adverse implications for infarct size and future heart failure risk. The consequently reduced access to acute revascularization and secondary prevention medications are expected to contribute importantly to excess acute cardiovascular deaths in the community, as reported by Wu and colleagues.[13]

Further reports indicate that there was, indeed, a significant drop in percutaneous coronary intervention (PCI) activity in the early stages of the pandemic, with Kwok and colleagues[20] demonstrating a 49% reduction in PCI procedures performed in England during the first wave of COVID-19 (March 2020), compared with prepandemic levels. Although (as expected) the greatest decline was in elective PCIs for stable coronary artery disease (−66%), PCIs for non-ST elevation myocardial infarctions (NSTEMI) or unstable angina (−45%) and ST-elevation MI (STEMI) also declined (−33%) substantially. In a national survey of interventional cardiology activity in Spain, Rodríguez-Leor et al.[21] also report significant reductions across all procedural activities, with 56% reduction in diagnostic coronary procedures, 48% reduction in PCIs for stable disease, and 40% reduction in PCI in STEMI. Consistently, Garcia and colleagues[22] reported a 38% reduction in PCI for STEMI across 9 hospitals in the US.

As may be expected from these observations, Rashid and colleagues[23] report a significant increase in the incidence of out-of-hospital cardiac arrests after the first wave of the pandemic in England (May 2020 vs February 2020). Ischemic disease is the most common precipitant of cardiac arrests. Disruptions in appropriate treatment of ACS as outlined previously predispose to greater and more prolonged ischemia, which may act as substrates for life-threatening ventricular tachyarrhythmias. Thus, the observed increase in out-of-hospital cardiac arrests by Rashid and colleagues[23] may reflect delays or failure to seek medical attention for ACSs.

A similar picture is seen in the context of acute stroke care. In a global registry of 187 stroke centers across 40 countries, Nogueira and colleagues[24] report a reduction in the number of stroke admissions, mechanical thrombectomy procedures, and intracranial hemorrhage admissions in association with the COVID-19 pandemic, independent of prepandemic admission/procedure volumes. Similarly, in a study of 19 EDs in the US, Uchino and colleagues[25] reported approximately 30% reduction in acute stroke presentations to the ED as well as a significant reduction in acute thrombolysis procedures suggesting delays in presentation. Indeed, in a study from China, Gu and colleagues[26] indicate significant prolongation of both pre and posthospital delays and significant reduction in the number of patients arriving within the time window for intravenous thrombolysis. These trends were consistent with those observed in the US by Schirmer and colleagues,[27] who also report significant prolongation of time to the presentation of acute ischemic strokes in the COVID-19 period compared with baseline prepandemic times. Poorer stroke outcomes in terms of death, disability, and recurrent stroke have been widely linked to increasing time from symptom onset to the initiation of stroke therapies such as thrombolysis and thrombectomy.[28] As such, the adverse public health impact of the described disruptions to stroke therapy is anticipated to be substantial.

Omissions and delays in care were also reported for other cardiovascular conditions with similar adverse prognostic consequences. Heart failure hospitalizations were notably reduced parallel to the first and second national lockdowns in the UK.[29] In a nationwide study, Shoaib and colleagues[30] demonstrate a decline in heart failure hospitalizations in England and Wales in March 2020 compared with preceding years. They further demonstrate a concordant increase in community heart failure deaths during this period.[30]

Overall existing evidence indicates reduced utilization of acute cardiovascular services with the resultant omission of key guideline-directed therapies and procedures, which likely explain excess cardiovascular mortality observed during the earlier phases of the pandemic. Individuals who survived acute untreated events are more likely to present in later postacute stages with complications or clinical decompensation and to have poorer outcomes than if they were treated appropriately at the outset. The longer-term impact of these missed care opportunities is yet to be fully appreciated, but likely will comprise an increase in both premature deaths and disability. In the clinical setting, it is important to remain vigilant to such potential late presentations of previously undetected acute events and to initiate appropriate therapies to minimize subsequent risks.

ELECTIVE ACTIVITY

As with acute care, there have been declines in elective procedures. While these procedures do not carry the same immediate urgency as the previously discussed acute conditions, substantial delays in their delivery lead to significantly poorer health outcomes. In this context, patients with severe aortic stenosis (AS) are a particularly at-risk group; these patients have an extremely poor prognosis in the absence of valvular intervention with a mortality rate of more than 50% at 2 years.[31] In a study of UK procedural registry data, Martin and colleagues[32] report a rapid and significant reduction in surgical aortic valve replacement (SAVR) and transcatheter aortic valve replacement (TAVR) procedures following the COVID-19 pandemic. The authors estimate that almost 5000 patients with severe aortic stenosis had not received appropriate procedural intervention in the months following the start of the pandemic (November to March 2020). These notable

treatment delays are expected to translate to poorer outcomes in this patient population, including higher risk of death and presentations with acute cardiovascular decompensation. Indeed, in a study of 22,876 patients with severe AS, Albassam and colleagues[33] report an association of greater wait time for valve intervention with higher risk of death and hospitalization for heart failure while on the waiting list. Thus, there is an urgent need to address strategies for service provision which may ameliorate these procedural backlog and treatment deficits.

The decline in elective work was observed across all cardiac interventions. In a study considering a wide range of cardiac procedures from the UK, Mohamed and colleagues[34] report a total deficit of more than 45,000 procedures over the COVID-19 period (March to May 2020) compared with previous years. In a study of over half a million patients referred for elective cardiovascular procedures from Canada, Tam and colleagues[35] report a significant decline in the number of coronary revascularization procedures performed during the pandemic compared with the prepandemic period. Importantly, the authors also observed an increased risk of all-cause death while waiting for coronary revascularization for referrals made during the pandemic. There was also evidence of change in the choice of procedural strategy. Among patients with left main coronary artery stenosis in the UK, there was an observation of both a reduction in revascularization procedures and greater use of PCI over coronary artery bypass grafting.[36]

The pandemic has also had a dramatic impact on cardiovascular imaging services with reduced activity due to the redeployment of staff and fewer referrals from both primary and secondary care. Cardiovascular imaging is central to the accurate diagnosis of many CVDs. In a survey of 909 centers covering 108 European centers, Williams and colleagues[37] report that total cardiac imaging reduced by 45% in March 2020 and by 69% in April 2020, compared with prepandemic levels. The authors demonstrate geographic variation in these trends with greater reductions observed in Southern European nations compared with elsewhere.[37] Consistent with these observations, in a study of 52 Italian centers, Dondi and colleagues[38] report a reduction in imaging volumes of 67% in March 2020% and 77% in April 2020, compared with the preceding year. These disruptions to clinical care raise concerns about large number of patients with delayed or missed diagnoses and the potential adverse impact of this on long-term risk of cardiovascular morbidity and mortality.

IMPACT ON PRIMARY CARE

The adverse impact of COVID-19 has extended to primary care, the key setting for primary prevention strategies and management of patients with stable chronic cardiovascular diseases. A UK report from NHS Digital,[39] indicated a near 30% reduction in appointments recorded in general practice systems in mid-March 2020, compared with prepandemic averages. In an analysis of nationwide general practice prescribing trends, Dale and Takhar and colleagues[40] demonstrate a reduction of incident use of antihypertensive and lipid-lowering medications in early 2021 compared with prepandemic levels in 2019. The authors estimate that the undertreatment of hypertension alone, is likely to result in 13,659 preventable cardiovascular events including 2281 additional myocardial infarctions and 3474 additional strokes.[40] In a study of more than 600,000 UK patients, Carr and colleagues[41] report a near 50% reduction in the measurement of blood pressure in general practice and 22% reduction in the prescription of new antihypertensive medications during the first year of the COVID-19 pandemic. An earlier nationwide study of patients with type 2 diabetes in the UK demonstrated a 31% reduction in glycated hemoglobin A1c (HbA1c) testing, 20% reduction in starting new metformin prescriptions, and 5% reduction in the initiation of insulin therapy.[42] These missed diagnosis and treatment optimization opportunities are concerning and have significant and sustained implications for population cardiovascular health. There is a need for dedicated efforts to address missed opportunities for primary and secondary prevention to alleviate the future population burden of cardiovascular disease.

INEQUITIES OF CARDIOVASCULAR CARE

The COVID-19 pandemic has highlighted the impact of social inequalities on health. Black Asian and Minority Ethnic (BAME) communities experienced higher infection and mortality related to COVID-19 compared with the White population.[43–48] Geography, deprivation, occupation, living arrangements, and health conditions such as cardiovascular disease and vascular risk factors account for some, but not all, of the excess mortality risk of COVID-19 in BAME populations.[46,49] As well as experiencing more severe outcomes from COVID-19, BAME cohorts also had disproportionately poorer cardiovascular outcomes during the pandemic. For instance, Kwok and colleagues[20] report the decline in PCI procedures to be more marked among patients with BAME, while Rashid and colleagues[23] found that BAME individuals were more likely to suffer out of hospital cardiac arrest during the pandemic. In a multisource linked cohort study, Rashid and colleagues[50] demonstrate that BAME individuals with acute myocardial infarction were less likely to receive guideline-directed therapies and had higher early mortality than White ethnicities, and, importantly, that these disparities seemed wider during the COVID-19 period compared with the prepandemic period. These poorer health experiences also extended to women and those from a more deprived background. For instance, Carr and colleagues[41] found that individuals with the highest levels of socio-economic deprivation experienced the greatest decline in general practice health checks for key cardiovascular risk factors. Similarly, Hartnett and colleagues[2] report a significant decline in ED visits of 42% during the early pandemic period and found that the steepest decreases were among women. These social inequalities were further exacerbated by the economic impact of the pandemic, which also disproportionately affected the most vulnerable in society. In a study including 27 European countries, Jiskrova and colleagues[3] report that job losses during the pandemic were significantly more likely among women, those with lower educational level, and lower household income.

Social and economic disadvantage are key determinants of health outcomes. The disproportionate impact of the pandemic on the most vulnerable in society mirrors the effect of other catastrophic natural disasters, where, consistently, the most devastating impacts are experienced by communities who are already disadvantaged and underserved.[51] COVID-19 has highlighted social inequalities and emphasized the urgent need for dedicated interventions to prevent and manage ill health in the most vulnerable populations. There is a need for high-quality data to understand the social and health care needs of deprived groups and to permit the development and tracking of appropriately targeted strategies by policy makers and health care professionals.

SUMMARY

The COVID-19 pandemic has adversely disrupted cardiovascular care across key areas of health care delivery including acute and chronic disease management and preventive interventions. The reduction in access to guideline-directed therapies and procedures in the acute setting has likely driven early observations of excess cardiovascular disease mortality. The substantial decline in elective cardiovascular procedures and significantly related backlog, if not promptly addressed, is expected to translate into excess death and disability in the medium term. Meanwhile, treatment deficits in primary and secondary disease prevention are expected to have a wider longer term impact in adversely impacting population cardiovascular health. The pandemic has shone a light on health care inequalities, which have been observed both in direct relation to COVID-19 and in the context of cardiovascular care during the pandemic. There is a need for concerted efforts from policy makers and clinicians to identify and actively address the deficits in cardiovascular health care resulting from the pandemic.

CLINICS CARE POINTS

- Health care professionals should remain vigilant to late presentations of acute cardiovascular conditions such as acute myocardial infarction and stroke, with a view to prompt the initiation of guideline-direct therapies to minimize subsequent cardiovascular risk.
- There is an urgent need for service planning to ensure the backlog of elective procedures, such as coronary revascularization, TAVR and SAVR, are addressed to prevent avoidable death and disability.
- Directed strategies in primary care to identify treatment deficits in primary and secondary cardiovascular prevention are strongly recommended to ensure the optimization of population cardiovascular health in the longer term.
- The pandemic has highlighted disproportionate adverse health outcomes experienced by BAME and deprived populations. There is a need for comprehensive high-quality data to better understand the specific health care needs of these communities. The reduction of health care inequalities requires directed efforts in multiple areas of health and social care and cohesive action from policy makers and health care professionals.

DISCLOSURE

Z. Raisi-Estabragh recognizes the National Institute for Health Research (NIHR) Integrated Academic Training program which supports her Academic Clinical Lectureship post and was also supported by British Heart Foundation Clinical Research Training Fellowship No. FS/17/81/33,318. M.A. Mamas has no disclosures.

REFERENCES

1. Ferraro CF, Findlater L, Morbey R, et al. Describing the indirect impact of COVID-19 on healthcare utilisation using syndromic surveillance systems. BMC Public Health 2021;21(1):1–11.
2. Hartnett KP, Kite-Powell A, DeVies J, et al. Impact of the COVID-19 pandemic on emergency department visits — United States, January 1, 2019–may 30, 2020. MMWR Morb Mortal Wkly Rep 2022;69(23):699–704.
3. Ksinan Jiskrova G, Bobák M, Pikhart H, et al. Job loss and lower healthcare utilisation due to COVID-19 among older adults across 27 European countries. J Epidemiol Community Health 2021;75(11):1078–83.
4. Xiao H, Dai X, Wagenaar BH, et al. The impact of the COVID-19 pandemic on health services utilization in China: time-series analyses for 2016–2020. Lancet Reg Heal - West Pac 2021;9:100122. https://doi.org/10.1016/J.LANWPC.2021.100122/ATTACHMENT/34CB8D18-1421-400E-BB7D-E7B00030A77D/MMC2.
5. Ahn S, Kim S, Koh K. Associations of the COVID-19 pandemic with older individuals' healthcare utilization and self-reported health status: a longitudinal analysis from Singapore. BMC Heal Serv Res 2022;22(1):1–8.
6. Chou Y, Yen Y, Chu D, et al. Impact of the COVID-19 pandemic on emergency healthcare utilization: a cohort study. Eur J Public Health 2021;31(December 2020):i352.
7. Roth GA, Mensah GA, Johnson CO, et al. Global burden of cardiovascular diseases and risk factors, 1990–2019. J Am Coll Cardiol 2020;76(25):2982–3021.
8. Islam N, Jdanov DA, Shkolnikov VM, et al. Effects of covid-19 pandemic on life expectancy and premature mortality in 2020: time series analysis in 37 countries. BMJ 2021;375:e066768.
9. Kontopantelis E, Mamas MA, Deanfield J, et al. Excess mortality in England and Wales during the first wave of the COVID-19 pandemic 2021;75(3):213–23.
10. Bae SA, Kim SR, Kim MN, et al. Impact of cardiovascular disease and risk factors on fatal outcomes in patients with COVID-19 according to age: a systematic review and meta-analysis. Heart 2021;107(5):373–80.
11. Kong KA, Jung S, Yu M, et al. Association between cardiovascular risk factors and the Severity of coronavirus disease 2019: nationwide Epidemiological study in Korea. Front Cardiovasc Med 2021;0:1066. https://doi.org/10.3389/FCVM.2021.732518.
12. Raisi-Estabragh Z, McCracken C, Cooper J, et al. Adverse cardiovascular magnetic resonance phenotypes are associated with greater likelihood of

incident coronavirus disease 2019: findings from the UK Biobank. Aging Clin Exp Res 2021;33(4): 1133–44.

13. Wu J, Mamas MA, Mohamed MO, et al. Place and causes of acute cardiovascular mortality during the COVID-19 pandemic. Heart 2021;107(2): 113–9.

14. Dreyer H, De Oliveira K, Lalloo V, et al. A qualitative study of COVID-19 related reasons for delayed presentation of patients with chest pain during the COVID-19 pandemic. Afr J Emerg Med 2022;12(1): 34–8.

15. Mafham MM, Spata E, Goldacre R, et al. COVID-19 pandemic and admission rates for and management of acute coronary syndromes in England. Lancet 2020;396(10248):381–9.

16. Braiteh N, Rehman W ur, Alom M, et al. Decrease in acute coronary syndrome presentations during the COVID-19 pandemic in upstate New York. Am Heart J 2020;226:147–51.

17. Nils P, Iglesias Juan F, Florian R, et al. Impact of the COVID-19 pandemic on acute coronary syndromes. Swiss Med Wkly 2020;150(51):1–8.

18. Eckner D, Hofmann EM, Ademaj F, et al. Differences in the treatment of acute coronary syndrome in the pre-COVID and COVID Era: an analysis from two German high-Volume Centers. J Cardiovasc Dev Dis 2021;8(11):145.

19. Aldujeli A, Hamadeh A, Briedis K, et al. Delays in presentation in patients with acute myocardial infarction during the COVID-19 pandemic. Cardiol Res 2020;11(6):386–91.

20. Kwok CS, Gale CP, Curzen N, et al. Impact of the COVID-19 pandemic on percutaneous coronary intervention in England: Insights from the british cardiovascular intervention society pci database cohort. Circ Cardiovasc Interv 2020; 210–21.

21. Rodriguez-Leor O, Cid-Alvarez B, Ojeda S, et al. Impact of the COVID-19 pandemic on interventional cardiology activity in Spain. REC Interv Cardiol 2020;2(2):82–9.

22. Garcia S, Albaghdadi MS, Meraj PM, et al. Reduction in ST-Segment elevation cardiac Catheterization Laboratory Activations in the United States during COVID-19 pandemic. J Am Coll Cardiol 2020; 75(22):2871–2.

23. Rashid M, Gale CP, Curzen N, et al. Impact of coronavirus disease 2019 pandemic on the incidence and management of out-of-hospital cardiac arrest in patients presenting with acute myocardial infarction in England. J Am Heart Assoc 2020;9(22). https://doi.org/10.1161/JAHA.120.018379.

24. Nogueira RG, Abdalkader M, Qureshi MM, et al. Global impact of COVID-19 on stroke care. Int J Stroke 2021;16(5):573–84.

25. Uchino K, Kolikonda MK, Brown D, et al. Decline in stroke presentations during COVID-19 Surge. Stroke 2020;51(8):2544–7.

26. Gu S, Dai Z, Shen H, et al. Delayed stroke treatment during COVID-19 pandemic in China. Cerebrovasc Dis 2021;50(6):715–21.

27. Schirmer CM, Ringer AJ, Arthur AS, et al. Delayed presentation of acute ischemic strokes during the COVID-19 crisis. J Neurointerv Surg 2020;12(7): 639–42.

28. Yafasova A, Fosbøl EL, Johnsen SP, et al. Time to thrombolysis and long-term outcomes in patients with acute ischemic stroke: a nationwide study. Stroke 2021;52:1724–32.

29. Wu J, Mamas MA, de Belder MA, et al. Second decline in admissions with heart failure and myocardial infarction during the COVID-19 pandemic. J Am Coll Cardiol 2021;77(8):1141–3.

30. Shoaib A, Van Spall HGC, Wu J, et al. Substantial decline in hospital admissions for heart failure accompanied by increased community mortality during COVID-19 pandemic. Eur Hear J - Qual Care Clin Outcomes 2021;7(4):378–87.

31. Vahanian A, Beyersdorf F, Praz F, et al. 2021 ESC/EACTS Guidelines for the management of valvular heart disease. Eur Heart J 2022;43(7):561–632.

32. Martin GP, Curzen N, Goodwin AT, et al. Indirect impact of the COVID-19 pandemic on activity and outcomes of transcatheter and surgical treatment of aortic stenosis in England. Circ Cardiovasc Interv 2021;14(5):e010413.

33. Albassam O, Henning KA, Qiu F, et al. Increasing wait-time mortality for severe aortic stenosis. Circ Cardiovasc Interv 2020;13(11):278–88.

34. Mohamed MO, Banerjee A, Clarke S, et al. Impact of COVID-19 on cardiac procedure activity in England and associated 30-day mortality. Eur Hear J - Qual Care Clin Outcomes 2021;7(3):247–56.

35. Tam DY, Qiu F, Manoragavan R, et al. The impact of the COVID-19 pandemic on cardiac procedure wait list mortality in Ontario, Canada. Can J Cardiol 2021; 37(10):1547–54.

36. Mohamed MO, Curzen N, de Belder M, et al. Revascularisation strategies in patients with significant left main coronary disease during the COVID-19 pandemic. Catheter Cardiovasc Interv 2021;98(7): 1252–61.

37. Williams MC, Shaw L, Hirschfeld CB, et al. Impact of COVID-19 on the imaging diagnosis of cardiac disease in Europe. Open Hear 2021;8(2):e001681.

38. Dondi M, Milan E, Pontone G, et al. Reduction of cardiac imaging tests during the COVID-19 pandemic: the case of Italy. Findings from the IAEA Non-invasive Cardiology Protocol Survey on COVID-19 (INCAPS COVID). Int J Cardiol 2021;341(January): 100–6.

39. Appointments in general practice - March 2020 - NHS Digital. Available at: https://digital.nhs.uk/data-and-information/publications/statistical/appointments-in-general-practice/march-2020#. Accessed January 5, 2022.

40. Dale CE, Takhar R, Carragher R, et al. The adverse impact of COVID-19 pandemic on cardiovascular disease prevention and management in England , Scotland and Wales : a population-scale descriptive analysis of trends in medication data. medRxiv Prepr 2022;1–41. https://doi.org/10.1101/2021.12.31.21268587.

41. Carr MJ, Wright Alison K, Leelarathna L, et al. Impact of COVID-19 restrictions on diabetes health checks and prescribing for people with type 2 diabetes: a UK-wide cohort study involving 618 161 people in primary care. BMJ Qual Saf 2021;0. https://doi.org/10.1136/BMJQS-2021-013613. bmjqs-2021-013613.

42. Carr MJ, Wright AK, Leelarathna L, et al. Impact of COVID-19 on diagnoses, monitoring, and mortality in people with type 2 diabetes in the UK. Lancet Diabetes Endocrinol 2021;9(7):413–5.

43. Morales DR, Ali SN. COVID-19 and disparities affecting ethnic minorities. Lancet 2021; 397(10286):1684–5.

44. Mathur R, Rentsch CT, Morton CE, et al. Ethnic differences in SARS-CoV-2 infection and COVID-19-related hospitalisation, intensive care unit admission, and death in 17 million adults in England: an observational cohort study using the OpenSAFELY platform. Lancet 2021;397(10286):1711–24.

45. COVID-19 takes unequal toll on immigrants in Nordic region. Available at: https://uk.reuters.com/article/uk-health-coronavirus-norway-immigrants/covid-19-takes-unequal-toll-on-immigrants-in-nordic-region-idUKKCN2260Y2. Accessed May 24, 2020.

46. Office for national Statistics- coronavirus (COVID-19) related deaths by ethnic group , England and Wales: 2 March 2020 to 10 April 2020. 2020. Available at: https://www.ons.gov.uk/peoplepopulationandcommunity/birthsdeathsandmarriages/deaths/articles/coronavirusrelateddeathsbyethnicgroupenglandandwales/2march2020to10april2020.

47. City of Chicago: Latest data. Available at: https://www.chicago.gov/city/en/sites/covid-19/home/latest-data/2020-04-21.html. Accessed May 24, 2020.

48. Raisi-Estabragh Z, McCracken C, Ardissino M, et al. Renin-angiotensin-aldosterone system Blockers are not associated with coronavirus disease 2019 (COVID-19) Hospitalization: study of 1,439 UK Biobank cases. Front Cardiovasc Med 2020;7(July):1–8.

49. Raisi-Estabragh Z, McCracken C, Bethell MS, et al. Greater risk of severe COVID-19 in Black, Asian and Minority Ethnic populations is not explained by cardiometabolic, socioeconomic or behavioural factors, or by 25(OH)-vitamin D status: study of 1326 cases from the UK Biobank. J Public Health (Bangkok) 2020;42(3):451–60.

50. Rashid M, Timmis A, Kinnaird T, et al. Racial differences in management and outcomes of acute myocardial infarction during COVID-19 pandemic. Heart 2021;107(9):734–40.

51. Ferdinand KC. Public health and Hurricane Katrina: lessons learned and what we can do now. J Natl Med Assoc 2006;98(2):271–4. Available at: https://pubmed.ncbi.nlm.nih.gov/16708514/. Accessed January 26, 2022.

Moving?

Make sure your subscription moves with you!

To notify us of your new address, find your **Clinics Account Number** (located on your mailing label above your name), and contact customer service at:

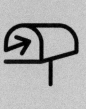

Email: journalscustomerservice-usa@elsevier.com

800-654-2452 (subscribers in the U.S. & Canada)
314-447-8871 (subscribers outside of the U.S. & Canada)

Fax number: 314-447-8029

Elsevier Health Sciences Division
Subscription Customer Service
3251 Riverport Lane
Maryland Heights, MO 63043

ELSEVIER

Printed and bound by CPI Group (UK) Ltd, Croydon, CR0 4YY

03/10/2024

01040363-0010